These materials are intended to provide assistance to the user as a reference tool. While every effort has been made to ensure the accuracy of the recommendations made herein, these materials are not intended to be a substitute for professional medical advice or treatment or the exercise of professional judgment in any given situation. Rather, these materials are intended only for general informational purposes. They reflect the best judgment of the editors and contributors as of the date of this publication and are subject to change. The content set forth in these materials should not be construed as the sole basis for the user's own medical judgments or decisions.

UNDER NO CIRCUMSTANCES WILL ISOQOL, ITS AFFILIATES OR ANY OF THEIR RESPECTIVE DIRECTORS, OFFICERS, MEMBERS, EMPLOYEES OR AGENTS, OR OTHERWISE ANY EDITOR OR CONTRIBUTOR TO THESE MATERIALS BE RESPONSIBLE OR LIABLE TO ANY USER OR OTHER ENTITY FOR ANY DIRECT, COMPENSATORY, INDIRECT, INCIDENTAL, CONSEQUENTIAL (INCLUDING LOST PROFITS OR LOST BUSINESS OPPORTUNITIES), SPECIAL, EXEMPLARY OR PUNITIVE DAMAGES THAT RESULT FROM OR RELATE IN ANY MANNER WHATSOEVER TO (1) USE OF THESE MATERIALS OR RELIANCE ON THE CONTENT THEREOF, OR (2) ERRORS, INACCURACIES, OMISSIONS, DEFECTS, UNTIMELINESS, SECURITY BREACHES OR ANY OTHER FAILURE TO PERFORM BY ISOQOL, ITS AFFILIATES OR ANY EDITOR OR CONTRIBUTOR HERETO.

Send comments to Colleen Pedersen, Executive Director, ISOQOL, at info@isoqol.org

QUALITY OF LIFE (QOL)

A term often used erroneously to refer to health-related quality of life or health status, but is broader than just health and includes components of material comforts, health and personal safety, relationships, learning, creative expression, opportunity to help and encourage others, participation in public affairs, socializing, and leisure. The WHO has defined quality of life as individuals' perception of their position in life in the context of the culture in which they live and in relation to their goals, expectations, standards and concerns. In the context of health research, quality of life goes beyond a description of health status, but rather is a reflection of the way that people perceive and react to their health status and to other, nonmedical aspects of their lives. According to Aristotle, quality of life would be the best kind of life, the happiest life, which is the life of virtue comprising: (i) intellectual or theoretical contemplation including scientific activity, considered the primary form of happiness; and (ii) practical or moral virtue including courage, moderation, generosity, and justice, the secondary form of happiness. In a modern context this would imply that one needs to think or contemplate aspects of life engagement and then act in a moral way or, in other words, be both smart and nice.

OUTCOME

In the context of health, an aspect of an individual's physical, emotional, mental or social health that is expected to change owing to a deliberate intervention or to vary in the presence of another personal, health or environmental factor. Kerr White coined the term the 5D's for health outcomes (death, disease, discomfort, disability, dissatisfaction). These have been updated to mortality (death), morbidity (disease), disability, dissatisfaction (with the process or the outcome), and cost (or the 6D, destitution which could be of the person or the health care system).

ISOQOL

Dictionary of Quality of Life and Health Outcomes Measurement

August 2015

Editor

Nancy Mayo, BSc(PT), MSc, PhD

James McGill Professor

Department of Medicine

School of Physical and Occupational Therapy

McGill University

Division of Clinical Epidemiology

Division of Geriatrics

McGill University Health Center

Dictionary Team (ABC order):

Sara Ahmed, David Andrich, Ruth Barclay, Skye Barbic, Susan Bartlett, David Bronstein, Cheryl Coon, Nandini Dendukuri, Diane Fairclough, Cindy Gross, Cicely Kerr, Ayse Kuspinar, **Carolina Moriello (Production Assistant),** Donald Patrick, Simon Pickard, Jacky Reid, Lena Ring, Ana Maria Rodriguez, Alicia Rosenzveig, Jennifer C Samp, Rick Sawatzky, Susan Scott, Lesley Wiseman, Jiameng Xu

Funding:

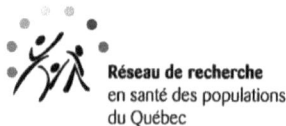

Réseau de recherche
en santé des populations
du Québec

INTRODUCTION

The idea of creating a dictionary of terms used in our field arose out of the Uruguay meeting in 2008. The stimulus came from an encounter with a discouraged student who had just realized that, although seasoned members of our society distinguished between quality of life and health-related quality of life (health and health status, a patient-reported outcome and a directly measured outcome), novices and researchers from other fields did not. I well remembered my years as a student in Epidemiology, another field replete with terms not well used by "outsiders", having Last's Dictionary of Epidemiology as an invaluable resource. Why not have such a resource for people working in the field of quality of life and health outcomes? This idea was enthusiastically received by the Board of Directors in 2009 and an initial call for contributors led us to a core Dictionary Team; others soon joined or were recruited.

In our initial enthusiasm, we developed a concept map to sketch out the areas where there was a need for consistent and correct terminology. We added terms to the concepts. We had other grandiose ideas as well. However, the reality of undertaking such a project with no dedicated resources soon hit and progress did not outpace a snail. However, all good ideas often just need time and some luck. In 2010, we had the opportunity to apply for a small amount of funding from the Quebec provincial government's Public Health Network dedicated for scholarly works. Armed with $5000 and a dedicated definition hounder (C Moriello), the Dictionary project took on new life.

Another chance encounter also helped considerably when I discovered, in June 2011, the Dictionary Society of North America which has over 400 members worldwide, a huge amount of knowledge, and a t-shirt. I now know that our group is writing a "vocabulary for a vertical audience" although it will be marketed as a "Dictionary". This will not be just any Dictionary and definitely not the Devil's Dictionary.

> Dictionary, n., *A malevolent literary device for cramping the growth of a language and making it hard and inelastic. This dictionary, however, is a most useful work.*
> —Ambrose Bierce, The Devil's Dictionary.

Along the way I discovered a "best-practice guideline" about definitions[1]. Interestingly, this is a field where "plagiarism" is acceptable – that is, if the term already has a definition then do not reinvent the wheel. This is because definitions are essentially information, and information cannot be owned. However, if a "lexicographer" cannot improve on the definition, she should give up her job. So as a first time "lexicographer", I attempted to make the definitions fit with the perspective of health outcomes measurement and make sense to readers. In other words, I attempted to assist the reader to visualize how a term is used or applied. Hence, Editor's prerogative was used to give concrete examples. As this is a "vocabulary" the definitions reflect the usage in quality of life and health outcomes measurement rather than all usages. As the audience is "vertical", the definition has to have meaning for the novice user as well as being useful for the expert.

The Dictionary would have been finished earlier had not each ISOQOL conference provided me with new terms to define, and indeed this indicates to me that even though a version has been produced, this dictionary needs to be a living document with new terms added as our "lexicon" expands and as our research and quality of life experience grows.

I am very grateful to the ISOQOL membership who provided helpful suggestions to improve the dictionary. Notably, I learned that quality of life is not just a concept that applies to humans, and I was happy to add definitions related to animal quality of life.

Many thanks to all the team who are listed on the inside cover who helped launch the idea and sent in definitions. A special thanks goes to Carolina Moriello who did all the production in addition to helping edit many definitions; this would not have happened without her help, support and belief in the process and outcome. Brenda Lee and Isabel O'Connor were very helpful in typing out many definitions and proof reading. Colleen Pedersen from the management team at ISOQOL championed the final product and saw that it left my desk and got published. I also wish to thank the board members of ISOQOL who had the patience to see the project to the end and to endorse the final product. Finally, but not least, I thank the ISOQOL members who took the time to review the product and make helpful additions for the final product.

It has been an amazing experience for me and I learned a tremendous amount about terminology, expressing complex ideas simply, and the breadth and depth of our field. I would not have missed this opportunity for the world.

Nancy E. Mayo, BSc(PT), MSc, PhD (nancy.mayo@mcgill.ca)

A

ACCEPTABILITY

In the context of research or clinical care, this refers to the question of whether or not study participants or patients are willing to do what is being asked of them.[2]

ACCURACY

The degree of conformity to a recognized measurement standard; refers to measurement properties of biological entities (biopsies, assays etc.). In the context of measuring constructs, this refers to the relative lack of error. Where there is no gold standard or no true value, this term is confused with validity.[3-5]

ACQUIESCENCE BIAS/OBSEQUIOUSNESS BIAS

The tendency to give responses that are perceived to be the most agreeable or helpful in the research context; a particular type of acquiescence bias is when a respondent gives all positive responses; this person is called a "yea-sayer"; the opposite is a "nay-sayer".[4, 6]

ACTIVITY

In the context of health, this is execution of a task or action by an individual; the WHO within the ICF framework classifies activities as those related to learning and applying knowledge, general tasks and demands, communication, mobility, self-care, domestic life and interpersonal interactions and relationships.[7]

ACTIVITIES OF DAILY LIVING

Basic tasks needed for performing personal care primarily bathing, dressing, moving around the house and eating; these activities represent primary biological functions reflecting the adequacy of the organization of neurological and locomotor systems.[8]

ACTIVITY LIMITATION

Difficulties an individual may have in executing activities; difficulty can be in terms of capacity (difficulty executing a task in a testing situation) or performance (difficulty in the person's usual environment); terminology within the WHO's ICF framework.[7]

ADAPTIVE DESIGNS

In randomized trials or surveys with sampling, the method of allocation or subject selection is modified over the course of the study to achieve balance on important co-variates; choosing this design renders the statistical analysis more complex as the time varying allocation or sampler's probability has to be considered.[3]

ADAPTIVE TEST

A form of test where the examinee is presented with an item and answers the question or performs the task. The next item presented to the examinee depends on their answer or performance on the previous item. This process continues until the person's value on the latent trait has been estimated with a satisfactory standard error of measurement set by the test administrator, a pre-set number of items has been administered, or all relevant content has been covered. This process avoids having persons with more (or less) capacity or milder (or more severe) disease perform tests or answer questions that are not relevant to their level. This reduces the total number of items administered and avoids boredom for those with higher capacity and discouragement for those with lower capacity. In a computer adaptive test (CAT), the item sequence is generated by a series of rules and the examinee only sees the items selected by the program; in a paper adaptive test, all items are presented and the examinee is directed to the relevant subtests based on response pattern.[9]

ADHERENCE (to therapy)

The extent to which a person's behavior – taking medication, following a diet, and/or executing lifestyle changes corresponds with agreed recommendations from a health care provider.[10] In the past, the term compliance and adherence were used interchangeably to refer to patients' behaviour but now the term compliance is used in the context of health professionals' or researchers' behaviours with respect to guidelines or protocols.

ADMINISTRATIVE DATABASES

Databases storing information routinely collected for the purposes of managing a health-care system. They are valuable sources of data as they cover the entire (insured) population but the information they contain was not collected for research purposes and hence their use requires a considerable amount of data management and a good understanding of the system they represent.[3]

ADVANCED DIRECTIVES

Legal documents that inform the doctor and family what a person wants for future medical care or decision making should the person later become unable to make decisions for him or herself. This may include whether to start or when to stop life-sustaining treatments or who should take over decision making.[11]

ADVOCACY

Taking action to help people to say what they want, securing their rights, representing their interests, and obtaining services they need. Most effective when carried out by a person who is independent of the services being provided.[12]

AETIOLOGY/ETIOLOGY

See CAUSE

AFFECT

A feeling, mood, emotion, or desire, especially as it influences behavior or thoughts; a key part of the process of an organism's interaction with stimuli and one of the ABCs of psychology: affect, behaviour, cognition.[13, 14]

AGEISM

Discrimination against or unfair treatment of individuals on the basis of their age.[12]

AGREEABLENESS

Agreeableness is one of the "big five" personality traits, reflecting an orientation towards being likable, pleasant and harmonious in interpersonal relationships with others. Individuals high in agreeableness are often described as being kind, considerate and warm, and express greater responsiveness and regulation of negative emotions in their interactions with others.[15]

AGREEMENT

Degree of concordance between two or more raters; crude agreement is the proportion of ratings that agree over the total number of ratings. Kappa is an agreement statistic based on the ratio of observed agreement to that expected by chance.[16]

AKAIKE'S INFORMATION CRITERIA (AIC)

An index used in statistical modeling to choose between competing models. It is defined as -2Lm + 2m, where L is the maximized log-likelihood and m is the number of parameters in the model. The model with the lowest AIC is considered the best model.[3]

ALL SUBSETS REGRESSION

A form of regression analysis in which all possible models are considered and the "best" selected based on a value on an appropriate criterion, such as Mallow's Ck.[3]

ALPHA ERROR

Probability of making a type I error (i.e., of concluding the two treatments differ when in reality they do not).[17]

ANCHOR

In the context of measurement, it is an external criterion that is a well interpretable measure to determine what patients or their clinicians consider as important improvement or important deterioration.[18] When Visual Analogue Scales are used, anchors are the terms or values at the ends of the scale that anchor the range.

ANCHOR-BASED

A method used to estimate the Minimally Important Change (MIC), or Minimal Important Difference (MID). The observed scores on the measure being tested for MIC are mapped onto values on anchored clinical tests that are considered important. Anchor-based differences can be determined either cross-sectionally (differences between clinically-defined groups at one time point) or longitudinally (change in score of one group over time).[2] With a cross-sectional study, an anchor-based method can also be referred to as known groups or discriminant validity.

ANONYMIZED

Previously identifiable data that has been de-identified and for which a code or other link no longer exists. An investigator would not be able to link anonymized information back to a specific individual.[19]

ANONYMOUS

Data that were collected without identifiers and that were never linked to an individual; data that are de-identified using codes for individuals are not anonymous.[19]

APATHY

The word apathy originated from the Greek word "apathes" (παθής) which means "without feeling". The first entry of the word apathy in the Oxford English Dictionary is from 1603, where it is defined as "freedom from, or insensibility to, passion or feeling; passionless existence". The current Oxford Dictionary definition reflects a more modern understanding: "indifference to what is calculated to move feelings; or to excite interest or actions". Apathy is the term used to describe the negative side of motivation. When symptoms of lack of initiative, energy, persistence, and drive are observable in a person, he/she is identified as apathetic. Apathy can be a trait, usually characteristic of the individual (i.e. a history of lifelong passivity, low role activity, low self-esteem, and low life satisfaction). Or apathy can be a state arising from a temporary adaptation to major changes in life (e.g. personal tragedy, natural catastrophe, social loss, and environmental deprivation). There is also a movement to declare apathy as a syndrome with a specific set of diagnostic criteria.[21] Apathy as a syndrome was first operationalized by Marin[21], and by Starkstein[22], however, today Robert et al.[24], reported on a consensus the apathy construct covers four domains: interest, action initiation, energy, and emotional response. In the context of health, apathy has been shown to be prevalent with neurological disease, and impacts on participation and engagement in meaningful activities. It has been measured using PROs as well as through family or health professional rating (ObsROs) of behaviours consistent with the domains of apathy.[20-23] See also MOTIVATION.

APPRAISAL

Psychological processes involved in rating personal experience with symptoms, functions, health, and quality of life; appraisal may affect future ratings of these outcomes if the person changes behaviours, priorities, or goals based on this appraisal. In the context of a clinical trial, appraisal can produce an impact on the magnitude of effect between two arms of an intervention study if the appraisal effect is differential across the different groups being compared: intervention, placebo, usual care, active control, as examples.[24]

AREA UNDER THE CURVE (AUC)

A useful way of summarizing the information from a series of measurements made on an individual over time, for example, those collected from a longitudinal study or for a dose-response curve. It is usually calculated by adding the areas under the curve between each pair of consecutive time points using, for example, the trapezium rule. This approximates calculating the area of a series of trapezoids (rectangles and triangles) and summing. This estimate best represents constructs that are always present in the individual to some degree but measured only periodically. For example, biological parameters such as blood sugar, cholesterol, lung capacity, or symptoms such as pain, fatigue, depression could be summarized over time using AUC.

Physical activity that happens sporadically would not be well represented.[3]

ASSISTIVE TECHNOLOGY

Technology used to help people maintain their independence, for example, using equipment and adaptations in their homes. Assistive technology includes innovations to assist with communication, equipment for people with a hearing disability, access for people with a visual disability, computer access for people with a learning disability, supporting people with dementia, linking housing and assistive technology, mobility, and wherever possible assessing physical ability to inform design. Telecare and telemedicine are applications within the assistive technology rubric as they enable individuals to be treated outside hospital settings and, by facilitating the work of physicians and community care teams, enable individuals with chronic illnesses or disabilities to live independently.[12]

ATTITUDE

Derived from an individual's values, an attitude typically reflects a tendency to react to certain events in certain ways and to approach or avoid those events that confirm or challenge the individual's values. Attitudes also affect individual beliefs and behaviour.[12]

ATTRIBUTE

Property or characteristic of an individual, such as eye colour. In measurement it refers to those characteristics which are measured with a high degree of certainty owing to the presence of a standard definition or test. For example, having a specific diagnosis would be an attribute. Attributes can also be assigned to treatments or medical devices.

ATTRITION

In the context of research, it is the dropping out of study participants over time; when this is differential between two comparison groups, such as in a randomized trial, this can lead to a bias, which must be corrected by using intention-to-treat analysis with some method of obtaining outcomes on all which may require statistically imputing the missing data.[5]

AUDIT

The examination or review of a practice, process, or performance in a systematic way to establish the extent to which they meet pre-determined criteria.[12]

AUTONOMY

The capacity to be one's own person, to live one's life according to reasons and motives that are taken as one's own and not the product of manipulative or distorting external forces. In the context of medicine it refers to the person's right to make their own decisions and is the basis of informed consent about care or engagement in research.[25]

AVATAR

In computing, an avatar is the graphical representation of the user or the user's alter ego or character. It may take either a three-dimensional form, as in games or virtual worlds, or a two-dimensional form as an icon in Internet forums and other online communities. In the context of disability, an avatar permits a person to take on an alter ego for the purposes of engaging in a virtual or online community.

B

BACK TRANSLATION

Translating back from the target language into the source language for the purposes of determining if the translation remains true to the intended meaning of the original document.[26]

BARRIER

A personal, environmental factor or an impairment or limitation that hinders performance or participation.[7]

BATTERY

In the context of health assessment, a series of tests or questionnaires designed to provide a comprehensive evaluation of a target construct and its associated constructs.

BAYESIAN STATISTIC

A method of statistical inference that requires the formulation of a probability distribution for the unknown parameters in a statistical model; the probability distribution is based on information external to the data (called prior distribution), such as the literature or pilot work. The prior distribution is then formally updated with the information in the observed data to obtain the posterior distribution of the unknown parameters. The prior distribution may be selected to reflect the investigator's subjective beliefs about the probability of the outcome, or it may be non-informative, depending on the context.[3, 5]

BAYESIAN INFORMATION CRITERION

An index used as an aid to choose between competing statistical models that is similar to Akaike's Information Criterion (AIC) but penalizes models of higher dimensionality (degrees of freedom) more than AIC. It is defined as $-2Lm + 2m\ln n$, where L is the maximized log-likelihood and m is the number of parameters in the model and n is the sample size, the model with the lowest BIC is considered the best model.[3]

BOOKMARKING

A method to identify cut-scores for symptom severity facilitated through the use of clinical vignettes representing graduated levels of symptom severity; clinicians and patients identify adjacent vignettes they judge to represent the threshold between two levels of severity for a given domain (e.g., threshold between a vignette that indicated "no problems" with a symptom and the adjacent one that represented "mild problems"). Cut-scores are defined as the mean location for each pair of threshold vignettes.[27]

BEREAVEMENT

Loss or separation from a loved one. Bereavement affects individuals in different ways as they grieve.[12]

BETA COEFFICIENT (β)

A regression coefficient that is standardized so as to allow for a direct comparison between explanatory variables as to their relative explanatory power for the response (outcome) variable. Calculated from the raw regression coefficients by multiplying them by the standard deviation of the corresponding explanatory variable.[3] This is also referred to as a STANDARDIZED REGRESSION COEFFICIENT which can be part of the output of a regression analysis but each particular statistical analysis package could have a different way of doing the standardization. For example in SAS (Statistical Analysis System), when using the ordinary least squares regression procedure (proc reg), the "stb" option for the model statement produces "standardized estimates" but these have been standardized by using the standard deviation of the outcome and of the explanatory variables, so the value is quite different than if standardization was done using the standard deviation of explanatory variables only.[28] See also REGRESSION COEFFICIENT

BETA ERROR

Probability of concluding that the groups do not differ when in reality they do differ (also called Type II error).[17]

BIAS

Systematic deviation of results or inferences from the truth. In the context of research, it arises from an error in the conception and design of the study, or in the collection, analysis, interpretation, reporting, publication, or review of data. Bias results in conclusions that are systematically, as opposed to randomly, different from the truth. In 1979, Sackett described 63 different kinds of bias.[6]

BLINDING

In the context of research, it is the process of keeping observers and/or subjects ignorant of the group to which the subjects belong; in an experiment blinding is with respect to group assignment; in the context of an observational study, blinding is respect to the population from which the subjects come. When both observer and subjects are kept ignorant, the study is referred to as a double-blind study, if the statistical analysis is also done in ignorance of the group to which subjects belong, the study is sometimes described as triple blind.[5]

BLOCKING

In the context of randomization, blocks of individuals (e.g. 2, 4, 6, 8, …) are randomized; this avoids an uneven allocation of subjects to groups and controls for secular trends.[29]

BODY FUNCTION

Within the WHO's ICF framework this refers to physiological functions of body systems (including psychological functions).[7]

BODY MASS INDEX (BMI)

An anthropometric measure of adiposity calculated as weight in kilograms divided by the square of height in meters (kg/m^2); BMI 18.5 is considered underweight, 18.5 to 24.9 is considered healthy weight, 25.0 to 29.9 is overweight; 30 to 39.9 is obese, and ≥ 40 is morbidly obese.[30]

BODY STRUCTURE

Within the WHO's ICF framework this refers to anatomical parts of the body such as organs, limbs and their components.[7]

BOOKMARKING

A method to identify cut-scores for symptom severity facilitated through the use of clinical vignettes representing graduated levels of symptom severity; clinicians and patients identify adjacent vignettes they judge to represent the threshold between two levels of severity for a given domain (e.g., threshold between a vignette that indicated "no problems" with a symptom and the adjacent one that represented "mild problems"). Cut-scores are defined as the mean location for each pair of threshold vignettes.[27]

BOOTSTRAP

A data-simulation method to obtain the variability and to provide confidence intervals for parameters in situations where these are difficult or impossible to obtain. The basic idea of the procedure involves sampling with replacement to produce random samples of size n from the original data (each of these is known as a bootstrap sample and each provides an estimate of the parameter of interest). Repeating the process a large number of times (1000 to 5000) provides the required information on the variability of the estimator and an approximate 95% confidence interval can be derived. Effect size (ratio of difference to standard deviation) and the regression parameter r^2 are examples of parameters for which confidence intervals can be obtained using bootstrapping. The term comes from the expression "to pull one's self up by the bootstraps".[3]

BURDEN OF CARE

In the context of health, it is the workload of health care and its impact on patient functioning and well-being, where "workload" consists of the demands placed on a patient by treatment for condition(s) and any associated health management strategies required (e.g. health monitoring, diet, exercise) and "impact" refers to the effect of treatment and self-care on a patient's behavioral, cognitive, physical, and psychosocial well-being.[31]

BURDEN OF DISEASE

A measurement of the gap between a population's current health and the optimal state where all people attain full life expectancy without suffering major ill-health.[32-34]

C

CAPACITY

Extent to which a task can be executed in a standard environment such as when tested in a clinical or laboratory setting; terminology from the WHO's ICF framework.[7]

CAPTURE-RECAPTURE METHOD

A method of estimating the size of a target population or a subset of this population that uses overlapping and presumably incomplete but intersecting sets of data about that population. The method originated in wildlife biology, where it relied on tagging and releasing captured animals and then recapturing them. The method was adopted in veterinary epidemiology and later in vital statistics (census taking) and epidemiology. If two independent sources or population estimates are available, with (a) cases found by both, (b) cases found only by the first source, or (c) cases found only by the second source, the maximum likelihood population estimate is the product of the total in each source divided by the total found in both sources, i.e., $(a + b) \times (a + c) / a$. If the two sources are positively (negatively) dependent, the result will be biased toward an underestimate (overestimate). If three or more sources are available, log-linear methods can sometimes be used to model the degrees of dependency among the sources. Although the capture-recapture methods have some limitations, they are useful to estimate numbers of cases and numbers at risk in elusive populations, such as homeless people and sex workers. See also SNOWBALL SAMPLING.[5]

CARE PATHWAY

Specifies treatment and care for a given condition based on nationally agreed guidelines, standards and protocols incorporating best practice and evidence-based guidelines. Care pathways, which map out the care journey an individual can expect, are multi-professional; cross organisational boundaries; and can act as a prompt for care. They provide a consistent standard of documentation which also provides the basis for ongoing audit.[12]

CARE PLAN

A personalised action plan that details the health and social care requirements a person needs based on their risks and measured impairments, limitations, and restriction; it should include details on the individual, the services to be provided, their carer(s) participation, the objectives of the plan, a review date, and consent from the assessed person to share the plan with the care team. The personalised care plan should also identify from the assessment the lifestyle and personal strengths of the person including their abilities, interests and wishes. The care plan should be printed in a suitable format for the individual and their carer(s).[12]

CAREGIVER

A parent, spouse, partner, child, relative or friend who provides regular and substantial unpaid care to someone who is disabled, severely ill or frail; care partner is often used to refer to caregivers who are spouses or play a spousal role.[12]

CASE-COHORT STUDY

A variant of the case-control study in which the controls are chosen from the same cohort as the cases regardless of their case status. Cases (persons with the disease or the outcome of interest) are identified and a sample of the entire starting cohort (regardless of their case status) forms the control group. This design provides an estimate of the risk ratio without any rare disease assumption.[5]

CASE-CONTROL STUDY

A study design that answers questions about factors that may prevent or cause a health condition or disease. Individuals with a particular condition or disease (the cases) are selected for comparison with a series of individuals without the condition or disease (the controls). Cases and controls are compared with respect to past attributes or exposures thought to be relevant to the development of the condition or disease under study. The underlying factors may either elevate or reduce the risk of disease, and a case-control study can quantify the alteration in risk associated with each factor individually and in combination. Case-control studies are often mislabelled. Use of the terms "cases" and "controls" are often a source of confusion for study designers and readers. Clinicians often use the expressions "cases" to refer to people with health conditions and "controls" to refer to healthy people who are recruited into studies to provide comparative data. In clinical situations, people with a condition (labeled cases) are compared to people without a condition (labeled controls) on current characteristics or on development of future outcomes. The key features of a case-control study are: (1) the question being answered is about etiology and not prognostication; (2) controls are matched to cases, they are not a convenient or parallel sample; (3) the exposure must precede in time the development of the condition defining a case and not be a consequence of being a case. For example, diet may change as a result of developing certain cancers, so dietary information would need to be collected prior to the person becoming a case. Case-control studies are referred to as retrospective designs because of the requirement that exposure must have occurred before the case became a case. A particular type of case-control study is a nested case control study in which there is an underlying cohort and cases and control arise from this cohort with the control being selected from among the pool of controls at the time the case became a case. For both types of case-control studies, more than one control can be selected per case and the control could become a case later on which makes sense if one considers a study of mortality: eventually all controls will become cases.[35-37]

CASE-CROSSOVER STUDY

An observational variant of the cross-over study used to study the acute effects of an exposure which triggers an event. Each subject serves as their own control in that the "case" time—the event—is compared to the control time for prevalence of the exposures hypothesized to trigger the event.[5]

CASE FATALITY RATE

Case fatality rate (percent) = # individuals dying during a specific period of time after disease onset or diagnosis / # of individuals with the specific disease.[17]

CASE MANAGEMENT

A process whereby a health professional actively manages and joins up care by offering, amongst others, continuity of care, coordination and a personalised care plan for vulnerable people most at risk because of numerous long term conditions and complex needs.[12]

CASE-ONLY STUDY

Similar to a case series often used in genetic epidemiology to assess relationships between environmental exposures and genotypes; cases with a particular disease or outcome and with a specific characteristic are compared to cases with the same disease but without the characteristic.[5]

CASE STUDY

A strategy for doing social inquiry that seeks to discern and pursue understanding of issues intrinsic to the case itself but where the cases are chosen and studied because they are thought to be instrumentally useful in furthering understanding of a particular problem issue, concept, etc.; the intent is to seek out both what is common about the case and what is unusual or particular. This strategy that is optimal when the inquiry revolves around the 'how' or 'why' in a contemporaneous and real-life context, when the researcher has little control over events being studied, and when it is desirable to use multiple sources of evidence.[38]

CATALYST

In the context of response shift this refers to health states or changes in health states, as well as other health-related events, treatment interventions, the vicarious experience of such events, and other events hypothesized to have an impact upon quality of life (life events).[39]

CAUSAL INDICATOR

In the context of testing the structural validity of an outcome measure such as one for HRQL or QOL using structural equation modeling (SEM), causal indicators, such as physical symptoms or negative side effects of treatment, are indicators related to the latent construct or factor; they are represented by reversal of the directional arrows so as to show that these indicators may be thought of as causing changes in the latent factors. In contrast, effect indicators are those domains of a QOL measure that may be impacted upon by change in the latent construct (QOL); psychological domains may be impacted upon by poor QOL and would be considered effect indicators.[40]

CAUSAL VARIABLE

In the context of the assessment of a latent construct such as quality of life, these are variables that are sufficient causes of change in the construct; that is, change in the causal variable is sufficient (but not necessary) to result in a change in the latent construct; symptoms would be causal variables for quality of life.[41]

CAUSE (NECESSARY)

A cause without which the outcome will not occur. Aristotle first identified four necessary causes of human action: material, efficient or moving, formal, and final. Material causes are akin to the lumber or other physical materials to build a house. In the context of quality of life, the domains of function could be debated as material causes. The builder, but more importantly the specific state that the builder is in, is the moving cause. In the context of quality of life several candidates emerge: hope, positive outlook, coping. The formal cause is akin to blueprints or plans, necessary to build a house. In the context of quality of life a candidate could be a plan and infrastructure to ensure needs are met. The final cause for Aristotle is the reason the house is being built. In the context of quality of life perhaps the final cause of quality of life is to achieve a degree of acceptance of the current condition or life situation, sometimes referred to as the "new normal".[42]

CAUSE (SUFFICIENT)

A cause which inevitably produces the effect; as a result, all persons with the cause will have the outcome. A sufficient cause acts on its own and no additional factors need to be present. Causes can be either or both necessary or sufficient. In the context of measuring a quality of life or PRO outcome, the presence of a symptom, for example, may be sufficient to cause a drop in quality of life, but it is not necessary because quality of life can drop because of other factors. Fayers warns against having sufficient causes as components of measures of quality of life because the presence just one cause will be sufficient to impact on quality of life leaving no room for other factors to have an effect.[42, 43]

CEILING EFFECT

See FLOOR AND CEILING EFFECTS.

CENSORED

In the context of a longitudinal study where time to reach an event or a particular health state is the outcome (survival analysis), people whose endpoint status cannot be determined because the study ended or the person was lost to follow-up are considered censored; people who reach the endpoint (termed a "failure" even if the event is positive) are classified as "failures"; all others are considered censored. To avoid bias, censoring should be independent of the variable understudy (exposure variable), termed the independent censoring assumption. For example, in a study of recovery of full participation post-surgery, if a person dies in a car crash before being assessed, they would be considered censored, and the independent censoring assumption would hold.[5]

CENTRAL LIMIT THEOREM (CLT)

A probability theorem about the sampling behaviour of a sample mean drawn from an underlying population with mean μ and standard deviation σ; samples of size n drawn from this population will have means that are distributed around μ and with standard deviation $\sigma/\text{sqrt}(n)$; the larger the n, the closer the distribution is to Gaussian (normal).[3]

CHANGE

In the context of measurement of health outcomes, change refers to the extent to which an individual's score evolves over time; this is to be distinguished from "difference" which refers to the dissimilarity of groups that are compared cross-sectionally[2]. There are many types of change that are relevant to health outcomes depending on whether change is considered from the person's or clinician's perspective[44]; this terminology has also evolved over time and different terms are used for essentially the same concept. When considering change, it is important to consider the concepts of change rather than solely their estimators.

1. MINIMAL CLINICALLY IMPORTANT DIFFERENCE (MCID). The smallest difference in score in the domain of interest which patients perceive as beneficial and which would mandate, in the absence of troublesome side effects and excessive cost, a change in the patient's management[45]. This term is best reserved for detecting between-group differences (see MID) and the term Minimal Important Change (MIC) for within-person change, although historically and even now the distinction is blurred. MCID and CID are outdated terms and are being replaced with MID and MIC.[46]

2. MINIMAL IMPORTANT DIFFERENCE (MID). The difference observed between groups that are known to differ on the construct of interest in an important way (e.g. by sex, age, or health status); the estimate is derived using known-groups methods.

3. MINIMAL IMPORTANT CHANGE (MIC). Smallest change in score in the domain of interest which patients perceive as important. For PROs, this should be considered from the patient's perspective, usually obtained by asking patients how much they have improved and calculating how much average change is observed for people saying they have changed "a little". For non-PRO measures both perspectives could be relevant. From the clinicians' perspective, a MIC may be one that indicates that a change in treatment may be warranted, or a change in the prognosis. In the context

of research, the MIC is used to estimate a sample size to provide adequate power to find the MIC statistically significant. MIC can be assessed using anchor based methods (change that is anchored in changes in an external criterion which can be from the patients' perspective or from changes in another measure) or distribution methods, such as change that ≥½SD.[47]

4. RESPONSIVENESS TO CHANGE. The consensus definition from the COSMIN panel is the ability of a test to detect change over time in the construct to be measured; this implies that change has occurred in that the magnitude of the change exceeds variation that can be attributed to chance or measurement error.[48] To illustrate the challenge in defining and estimating this concept, Terwee identified 25 definitions of responsiveness and 31 estimators (formulae).[49]

5. SENSITIVITY TO CHANGE. The ability of a test to measure change in the health state of the person regardless of whether it is meaningful to the decision maker; necessary but not sufficient conditions for responsiveness.[50]

6. SMALLEST DETECTABLE CHANGE (SDC). (also called Minimal Detectable Change) Change beyond measurement error which can be illustrated by change that falls outside the limits of agreement of the Bland and Altman plot, essentially change larger than ±1.96SD of change or larger than ±1.96 x √SEM (standard error of measurement). This is an indicator of how much scores can vary in stable patients.[2]

CHECKLIST

A series of items that may produce a score through simple aggregation. For example, in a questionnaire that asks patients about the presence of different physical symptoms, a checklist may be constructed to represent the number of problems that a patient reports. A checklist differs from an index in that a checklist is merely a compilation of items and may not have a psychometrically sound underpinning.[51]

CHEMOPREVENTION

The use of natural or laboratory-made substances to prevent cancer.[52]

CHRONIC CARE MODEL (CHRONIC DISEASE MODEL)

A comprehensive framework for the organization of healthcare to improve outcomes for people with chronic conditions. It comprises six elements: health care organization, community resources, self-management support, delivery system design, decision support, and a clinical information system. The aim of deploying this model in clinical care is to develop a productive interaction between the skilled health professional and the knowledgeable patient. This interaction is supported by clinical guidelines, information systems, and a local organization for case management. Patient education and behaviour change are key features of chronic disease management, which is enhanced by a self-management plan.[53]

CLASSICAL TEST THEORY

A measurement theory based on the premise that the raw score of a person on a test composed of multiple items is a function of the true score and random error; the error is the same for each person.[54]

CLINICAL OUTCOME ASSESSMENT

Any assessment that may be influenced by human choices, judgment, or motivation and may support either direct or indirect evidence of treatment benefit. Unlike biomarkers that rely completely on an automated process or algorithm, COAs depend on the implementation, interpretation, and reporting from a patient, a clinician, or an observer. The four types of COAs are patient-reported outcome (PRO) measures, clinician-reported outcome (ClinRO) measures, observer-reported outcome (ObsRO) measures, and performance outcome (PerfO) measures.[55]

CLINICAL PRACTICE GUIDELINES

Systematically defines statements to assist practitioner and patient decisions about appropriate health care for specific clinical circumstances.[52]

CLINICAL TRIAL

A formal study carried out according to a prospectively defined protocol that is intended to discover or verify the safety and effectiveness of procedures or deliberate interventions in humans; the intervention is often an innovation in treatment.[56]

CLINICALLY IMPORTANT DIFFERENCE

See CHANGE.

CLINICIAN-REPORTED OUTCOME (ClinRO or CRO)

In the context of an end-point for a study, a ClinRo or CRO is an outcome that is either observed by an expert such as a physician, other health professional, or trained individual (e.g., cure of infection and absence of lesions) or requiring interpretation by such expert (e.g., radiologic results and tumor response). ClinROs are completed by the expert using information about the patient.[57]

CLINIMETRICS

The term "clinimetrics" was introduced by Alvan R. Feinstein in 1982 to indicate a domain concerned with indexes, rating scales and other expressions that are used to describe or measure symptoms, physical signs, and other distinctly clinical phenomena in medicine. The purpose of clinimetric science was to provide an intellectual home for a number of clinical phenomena, which do not find room in the customary clinical taxonomy. Such phenomena include the types, severity and sequence of symptoms; rate of progression of illness, severity of comorbidity; problems of functional capacity; reasons for medical decisions; and many other aspects of daily life, such as well-being and distress.[58]

CLUSTER ANALYSIS

A set of methods for constructing a (hopefully) sensible and informative classification of an initially unclassified set of data, using the variable values observed on each individual. Essentially all such methods try to imitate what the eye-brain system does so well in two dimensions. For example, it is very simple to detect the presence of three clusters without making the meaning of the term 'cluster' explicit.[3]

CLUSTER RANDOMIZED TRIAL

A study of a deliberate intervention where the unit of randomization contains several or many individuals such as communities, worksites, hospitals, schools, or medical practices. Dependencies among cluster members must be considered when determining sample size and in the subsequent data analyses. Failure to adjust standard statistical methods for within-cluster dependencies will result in underpowered studies with spuriously elevated Type I errors.[59]

COCHRANE REVIEW

Cochrane Reviews are systematic reviews of research in healthcare and health policy that are published in the Cochrane Database of Systematic Reviews. There are three types of Cochrane Review: (1) Intervention reviews that assess the benefits and harms of interventions used in healthcare and health policy, (2) Diagnostic test accuracy reviews that assess how well a diagnostic test performs in diagnosing and detecting a particular disease, and (3) Methodology reviews address issues relevant to how systematic reviews and clinical trials are conducted and reported. Cochrane Reviews base their findings on the results of trials which meet certain quality criteria, as the most reliable studies will provide the best evidence for making decisions about health care. Authors of Cochrane Reviews apply methods which reduce the impact of bias across different parts of the review process, including: (i) identification of relevant studies from a number of different sources (including unpublished sources); (ii) selection of studies for inclusion and evaluation of their strengths and limitations on the basis of clear, predefined criteria; (iii) systematic collection of data; and (iv) appropriate synthesis of data.[59, 60]

COGNITIVE DEBRIEFING/COGNITIVE INTERVIEWING

Interviews to examine the cognitive processes employed by respondents as they go through the process of answering a given survey question. Essentially these interviews are designed to get at the what (meaning), how (decision process behind choosing a response), when (time period), why (reasoning in choosing a response), where (calibration decisions), and who (reference comparator) behind how an individual chose a response to an item. Techniques including "think aloud" while responding to the question, probing, and paraphrasing are used. The aim is to ensure that respondents interpret and respond to the question in the intended manner; this is a crucial step during the development phase of a PRO or survey questionnaire.[61-63] Also used in the translation process to ensure cross-cultural validity and other types of translation-related validities. Blair et al.[63] provide statistical information to determine how many cognitive interviews are required to identify the majority of problems with a survey instrument.

COGNITIVE RESERVE

See RESERVE.

COHEN'S KAPPA

See KAPPA.

COHORT MULTIPLE RANDOMIZED CONTROLLED DESIGN

A design in which a fully characterized cohort is followed over time providing rich observational data for modeling and understanding change in health outcomes; added to the cohort study are a set of trial protocols that target specific outcomes in sub-groups of the population that would benefit the most. People meeting intervention-specific criteria are randomly selected to receive an intervention and the rest of the eligible cohort members serve as controls, increasing power. This design is ideal for testing multiple interventions in one cohort as there is a common outcome strategy for all with fixed evaluation time points and harmonized strategies to ensure complete follow-up. In addition each intervention trial can have some degree of standardization in terms of responder-definition and statistical methodology making the total impact of the trials much greater than the sum of the individual trial components. Most importantly, all members of the cohort have the opportunity to receive one or more interventions, increasing engagement and reducing missing data.[64]

COHORT STUDY

A study in which the investigator selects a population composed of exposed individuals and non-exposed individuals and follows all to compare them on the cumulative incidence of an outcome, such as disease or event, or on the rate of occurrence of an outcome or event in which case time must be part of the denominator as in number of outcomes per unit of person-time.[17]

1. INCEPTION COHORT STUDY: A type of cohort study in which individuals are identified at an early and uniform point in the course of the health condition under study or before the health condition develops.[65] Certain health conditions lend themselves to the inception cohort approach because of a sudden or defined onset, such as stroke, myocardial infarction, accidents or injury. Studies of these types of conditions that do not use an inception cohort approach can introduce selection bias or survival bias in that the people entering the cohort are not representative of all the people at the inception of the health condition.

2. HISTORICAL (OR RETROSPECTIVE) COHORT STUDY: A comparison of exposed and non-exposed populations where exposure is ascertained from past records or from recalling past events and outcome (development or not of disease) is ascertained at the time the study is begun; the term historical cohort is preferred when the information on exposure in the past is obtained from historical data rather than recalled.[17]

3. PROSPECTIVE COHORT STUDY: A study that is used to identify causes of events or health conditions; the population is assembled at the beginning of the study and the subjects are followed concurrently through calendar time until the point at which the disease

develops or until study end; ; at the study end, the rate or risk of outcome in people with the factor under study is compared to the rate or risk of outcome in people without the factor; this type of study permits the counting of person-time in view and using this as the denominator for the estimates of rates. Although any study that follows people longitudinally over time is sometimes called a cohort study, a more correct term for these studies, when they are not population-based and not concerned with etiology but perhaps with prognosis, is a longitudinal study.[17]

COLD DECK

A method of replacing missing data by using external data sources such as from a previous data collection or a different data set; this and the term "hot deck" imputation are derived from the time when data was processed using computer punch cards; if existing data are used for missing values, the cards are not processed and hence the deck remains "cold".[66]

COMORBIDITY

Diseases that coexist in a person with an index condition but are neither the cause nor the consequence of the index condition. Comorbidity affects mortality, health resource utilization, admission and readmission to hospital, and health related quality of life (HRQL) or functional status.[5, 67]

COMORBIDITY INDEX

A weighted measure that, with conducting statistical analyses, will control for the potential influence of those illness on an outcome of interest. Indices include simple methods such as counting the number of health conditions, or methods based on diagnoses such as that developed by Charlson.[68]

COMMUNITY-DWELLING

A description of a population who is living in the community rather than in an institution.

COMPANIONSHIP SUPPORT

A type of social support involving the availability of persons with whom one can participate in social and leisure activities such as trips and parties, cultural activities (e.g., going to movies or museums), or recreational activities such as sporting events or hiking.[69]

COMPARATIVE EFFECTIVENESS RESEARCH (CER)

The generation and synthesis of evidence that compares the benefits and harms of alternative methods to prevent, diagnose, treat, and monitor a clinical condition or to improve the delivery of care. In the context of PRO research, when information is collected on outcomes that patients care about, beyond only survival and biomedical findings (which are often similar between treatments), the patient's experience can make the defining contribution to the comparison. The key elements of CER are (a) head-to-head comparisons of active treatments, (b) study populations typical of day-to-day clinical practice, and (c) a focus on evidence to inform care tailored to the characteristics of individual patients. A deliverable from CER is evidence as to what works best for whom and under what circumstances.[70]

COMPLIANCE

In the research context, this term refers to the extent to which the elements of a research protocol are followed by the investigators and the research subjects; for subjects compliance can be calculated as the percentage of instances that a study measure was completed divided by the total possible completion opportunities in a given study.

COMPOSITE

In the context of health outcomes, a composite outcome is one that is comprised of several outcomes which have been combined using a pre-defined algorithm; anyone who responds to or experiences one of the outcomes is considered to have responded to or experienced the composite.[3, 71, 72]

COMPUTER ADAPTIVE TESTING (CAT)

Form of adaptive testing in which an interactive computer presents test items to an individual, accepts and scores the item responses, chooses the next item based on the response, and terminates the test when an appropriate; use of a CAT increases efficiency as fewer items (50% to 80% fewer) need to be administered to obtain the same measurement quality as the conventional test; or better measurement quality can be obtained with the same number of items.[9] See also ADAPTIVE TEST.

COMPUTER ASSISTED INTERVIEW

A method of data collection with questions displayed on a computer and responses entered directly into a computer.[73]

CONCEPT

Global definition and demarcation of the subject of measurement.[18]

CONCEPT MAPPING

Specific, definable processes which can be used to organize thinking and to represent it for others to see. Generally the components of concept mapping are: (i) the processes or the steps followed to conduct the conceptualization; (ii) the perspective for the concept from the persons involved in the process; and (iii) the final representation form for the concept. Concept mapping involves generating the domain to conceptualize which are the set of initial entities such as thoughts, intuitions, ideas, theories or problems; structuring of the domain by defining or estimating the relationships between and among the entities; and representing the conceptual domain verbally, pictorially or mathematically.[74]

CONCEPTUAL FRAMEWORK

A model representing the relationships between the items and the construct to be measured, as in a reflective or formative model. A reflective conceptual model would be one where the construct is reflected by the items; a formative model is when the construct is the result of the items such that the items form or cause the construct. Anxiety is an example of construct based on a reflective model because anxiety is reflected in items relating to worrying thoughts, panic, or restlessness; if the construct changed, these items would change. Life stress is an example of a construct based on formative model as different life experiences "cause" stress and if the construct changed, the experiences themselves would not result.[18, 43]

CONCEPTUAL MODEL

In the context of health outcomes research, this is a theoretical model of how different constructs within a concept are related. Examples are the WHO-ICF model and the Wilson-Cleary Model.[18]

CONCORDANCE

See AGREEMENT.

CONCURRENT COHORT

See PROSPECTIVE COHORT.

CONCURRENT VALIDITY

A form of criterion validity when both the score for the measurement and the score for the gold standard are considered at the same time; often assessed using sensitivity and specificity.[18]

CONDITION SPECIFIC MEASURES

Outcomes that relate to symptoms associated with a disease or illness or to health situations (condition) that would not be classified as a disease or illness; examples include obesity, small-stature, disfigurement, menopause, pregnancy.[75]

CONFIDENCE INTERVAL

A range of values within which the value of that variable in the population is thought to lie with a specified probability.[76]

CONFIRMATORY FACTOR ANALYSIS (CFA)

A method to test whether a hypothesized factor structure of a questionnaire (based either on empirical data or on theory) is supported by actual data[18]; Structural equation modeling (SEM) techniques are used to test hypotheses about relationships between observed variables (items) and factors. A model must be specified a priori and formal tests of goodness of fit are used to confirm that the data fit the model; factor loadings measure how well the observed variables measure the latent construct.[77, 78]

CONFIRMATORY HYPOTHESIS

The hypothesis for which a particular study was designed and powered to test. It is distinguished from explanatory and exploratory hypotheses that may also be tested using data arising from the study.[79]

CONFOUNDING

In the context of a particular study, it is a variable that is associated both with the exposure (or explanatory variable) and with the outcome variable but is not in the causal pathway between exposure and outcome. In the context of quality of life research the association between hypothesized contributors (explanatory variables) and quality of life (outcome) may be confounded by variables that independently affect both, such as age, gender, environmental factors, for examples. If these are not considered in the study design the association can be biased. Five strategies are typically used to control for confounding; restriction of the sample to those without the factor, stratification with stratum specific analyses, matching, randomization (if possible), and analysis after using statistical adjustment.[42]

CONJOINT ANALYSIS

Rigorous method of eliciting preferences by allowing estimation of the relative importance of different aspects of health or of health care. The technique is based on the premises that any health state or service can be described by its characteristics (or attributes), and that the extent to which an individual values a health state or service depends on the levels of these characteristics. The characteristics are used to create realistic scenarios and preferences for the selected scenarios are elicited by using one of three methods: ranking, rating, or discrete choices. With ranking, respondents are asked to list the scenarios in order of preference. This method has not as yet been used in health care. The rating method requires the respondents to assign a score, of say 1 to 5, to each of the scenarios. For the discrete choice method, respondents are presented with a number of choices and, for each, asked to choose their preferred one. Possible responses include stating that either A or B is preferred, or responding on a five-point scale where 1 equals definitely prefer A and 5 equals definitely prefer B. Given that choices more closely resemble real life decisions, the discrete choice approach has been preferred in health care.[80]

CONSORT

Consolidated Standards of Reporting Trials encompasses various initiatives developed by the CONSORT Group to address problems related to inconsistent reporting of results from randomized controlled trials (RCTs). The CONSORT Statement is a minimum set of recommendations for reporting RCTs. The recommendations offer a standardized method to report trial findings, facilitating complete and transparent reporting, and aiding their critical appraisal and interpretation. Use of the CONSORT format is required for articles published in major biomedical journals.[81]

CONSTRUCT

An intangible, theoretical entity that will be operationalized into 1 or more items. Pain, anxiety and other symptoms are examples of constructs that can be described in many ways (e.g. frequency, intensity, duration, characteristics).[51]

CONSTRUCT VALIDITY

The degree to which the scores of a measure are consistent with hypotheses (for instance with regard to internal relationships, relationships to scores of other measures, or differences between relevant groups) based on the assumption that the measure validly quantifies the construct of interest.[46]

CONTENT

The degree to which (the items of) a measure looks as though they are an adequate reflection of the construct to be measured.[46]

CONTENT ANALYSIS

A generic name for a variety of means of initial analysis that involves comparing, contrasting, and categorizing a corpus of data derived from cultural artifacts (texts, documents, television programs, etc.) or events. Classical content analysis emphasises systematic, objective, and quantitative description of content derived from researcher–developed categories but now more contemporary forms of content analysis include both numeric and interpretive means of analysing data.[38]

CONTENT VALIDITY

The degree to which the content of an HR-PRO instrument is an adequate reflection of the construct to be measured[46]; it is reflected by the extent to which an instrument contains the relevant and important aspects of the content it intends to measure, and the content was derived by following best practices in measure development that involve concept elicitation and cognitive debriefing with patients.[55]

CONTEXT/CONTEXTUAL FACTORS

Group or macro-level variables that play a role in the determination of disease in populations.[82]

CONTINUITY OF CARE

Continuity is the degree to which a series of discrete healthcare events is experienced as coherent and connected and consistent with the patient's medical needs and personal context. It involves the relationship between a single practitioner and a patient that extends beyond specific episodes of illness or disease; its two key distinguishing elements are care of an individual patient, and care delivered over time.[83]

CONVERGENT VALIDITY

A type of construct validity in which specific hypotheses are tested regarding how the measure under study relates to related constructs as opposed to unrelated constructs (divergent validity).[18]

CORNER-STATE

In the context of the valuation of health states, a corner-state is the multi-dimensional health state where one item is at its worst level and all the other items are at the best levels.[84]

CORRELATION COEFFICIENT

Is an index that quantifies the strength of the linear relationship between two variables? The correlation coefficient can take values from -1 to +1, with 0 indicating no relationship (random pairing of values) and 1 indicating perfect relationship. A warning about using correlation to estimate inter-rater reliability is that one rater may consistently evaluate a sample of people lower than the other rater indicating little agreement, yet the correlation between the two raters will be very high, near 1.0.

There are different types of correlation coefficients depending on the nature and distribution of the variables to be correlated.[2, 5] One consideration in choosing which correlation coefficient to use is whether the data arise from variables with an underlying distribution that is *"perfectly precise, normally distributed, real numbers"* (PPNDRN) or the data arise from naturally discrete variables with 2 or more specific values. A second consideration is whether the PPNDRN variables are treated as continuous or have been categorized into 2 or more classes.[85, 86] The table below illustrates the match between the type of variable and the correlation coefficients.

		Variable B				
		PPNDRN			DISCRETE (NOMINAL)	
Variable A		CONTINUOUS	2 CLASSES	≥3 CLASSES	2 VALUES	≥3 VALUES
PPNDRD						
CONTINUOUS		Pearson (Spearman if ranks)	Biserial	Polyserial	Point-biserial	Point-polyserial
2 CLASSES			Tetrachoric	Rank-biserial	Phi	Kendall's W
≥3 CLASSES				Polychoric	Kendall's Tau	Kendall's W
DISCRETE (NOMINAL)						
2 VALUES					Phi	Kendall's W
≥3 VALUES						Kendall's W

1. PEARSON PRODUCT MOMENT: The most commonly used method of computing a correlation coefficient between variables that are PPNDRN and the data are continuous.

2. SPEARMAN: Is simply Pearson's product moment correlation between two variables in which the scores have been ranked and the ranks correlated.

3. BISERIAL: Both of the variables are PPNDRN; one retains its continuous nature and the other has been categorized to produce 2 classes. A biserial correlation would be used to correlate a measure of quality of life (continuous) with cognitive ability which is an underlying continuous construct but recorded as impaired or not.

4. POLYSERIAL: The extension of the biserial correlation but with three or more classes.

5. TETRACHORIC: Used when two PPNDRN variables have both been categorized to produce two classes. In the example for biserial correlation, the tetrachoric correlation would be used if the quality of life variable had been categorized into optimal and sub-optimal correlated.

6. POLYCHORIC: Is the extension of the tetrachoric but for two PPNDRN variables that have been categorized into three or more classes. For example, health perception, an underlying continuous construct, categorized into Excellent, Very good, Good, Fair and Poor (EVGGFP) correlated with cognitive ability categorized into three levels. Correlation between two variables measured on Likert Scales is another example of the use of the polychoric correlation. It is based on the assumption that the ordinal scoring arises from partitioning the range of some continuous normally distributed variables into categories; the correlation between the two unobserved continuous variables is what is of interest. This type of correlation has been used to assess rater agreement on ordinal variables; it generalizes to a latent trait model with more than two raters and provides a test of whether all raters have the same definition of the latent trait while simultaneously testing for equivalents of thresholds among

all raters. Now it is widely used in the context of evaluating the properties of ordinal rating scales using Rasch Analysis.

7. RANK BISERIAL: Is used when an ordinal variable of 3 or more classes is correlated with a variable with 2 classes.

8. POINT BISERIAL: Used in the case where one variable is PPNDRN and the continuous scale is retained and the other variable is naturally discrete with only two values. An example would be quality of life and gender.

9. POINT POLYSERIAL: Is the extension of the point biserial correlation but now one of the variables is naturally discrete with three or more levels, an example might be falls.

10. KENDALL'S TAU: Is when one variable representing 2 discrete (nominal) groups is correlated with another variable which is ordinal or ranks

11. KENDALL'S W: The extension of Kendall's Tau when one variable represents 3 or more discrete (nominal) groups and the other variable is ordinal or ranks.

12. PHI: A correlation between two variables that are discrete with only 2 categories or values, for example living in long term care or not and mortality in an older frail population.

COST-BENEFIT ANALYSIS

Cost-benefit Analysis (CBA) is an economic evaluation in which all costs and consequences of a program are expressed in the same units, usually money. CBA is used to compare costs and benefits across programs serving different patient groups, termed allocative efficiency. Even if some items of resource or benefit cannot be measured in monetary terms, they should not be excluded from the analysis.[30]

COST-EFFECTIVE ANALYSIS

Cost-effectiveness analysis (CEA) is one form of full economic evaluation where both the costs and consequences of health programmes or treatments are examined. Examples of effectiveness measures used in CEA are episode-free days, life-years gained, and percent reduction in an outcome of interest.[87]

COST-MINIMIZATION

Cost-Minimization Analysis (CMA) is an economic evaluation in which consequences of competing interventions are the same and in which only inputs that is, costs are taken into consideration. The aim is to decide the least costly way of achieving the same outcome.[30]

COST UTILITY ANALYSES

A form of economic analysis in which interventions which produce different consequences, in terms of both quantity and quality of life, are expressed as 'utilities'. These are measures which comprise both length of life and subjective levels of well-styembeing. The best known utility measure is the 'quality adjusted life year' or QALY. In this case, competing interventions are compared in terms of cost per utility (cost per QALY).[30] See also QUALITY ADJUSTED LIFE YEAR.

COX'S PROPORTIONAL HAZARD RATIO

A statistical method for analyzing survival data or any data where time to develop an outcome is under study. It assumes that the effect of study factors on the hazard rate (instantaneous rate of developing the outcome at a particular time) do not vary over time. It assesses the instantaneous probability that an individual who is well at a specific time will experience the outcome event at the next instant.[5]

CRITERION VALIDITY

The degree to which the scores of an instrument are an adequate reflection of a ''gold standard''.[46]

CRONBACH'S ALPHA

Cronbach's Alpha, also known as coefficient alpha, is a measure of the internal consistency of a set of items. Internal consistency is a form of reliability and, like other measures of reliability in classical test theory, Cronbach's alpha can be defined as an estimate of the ratio of true variance (variance due to the underlying construct) to total variance (true variance plus error) for a measure. When items are highly inter-correlated, the collection of items is assumed to strongly reflect the intended latent construct. A common formula for Cronbach's alpha is based on the average inter-item correlation (labeled ra) and k, the number of items in the scale: Alpha = kra/[1+ (k-1)ra]. The Kuder-Richardson formula 20 (KR-20) which measures internal consistency for scales with dichotomously scored items is computationally equivalent to Cronbach's alpha. Values should by higher than 0.7 but lower than 0.9.[77, 88]

CROSS-CULTURAL VALIDITY

The degree to which the performance of the items on a translated or culturally adapted index are an adequate reflection of the performance of the items of the original version of the index.[46]

CROSS-OVER DESIGN

Subjects are randomized to therapy "A" or therapy "B" and after being observed for a certain period of time on one therapy, they are switched to the other therapy.[17]

CROSS SECTIONAL STUDY

A study where both the exposure and outcome are determined simultaneously for each subject providing a snapshot of the population at a certain point in time; it is useful for estimating prevalence of an outcome, and associations between exposures and outcomes, but cannot be used to infer causality.[17]

CROSS-VALIDATION

See INTERNAL CROSS VALIDATION.

CRUDE AGREEMENT

The extent to which multiple ratings of an object agree exactly on how the object is to be classified.[16]

CULTURAL ADAPTATION

Process of adapting the content of a measure during the translation process to improve the cultural relevance of the content to the target culture. For example some activities like golf or curling are not common in all cultures so these activities would be replaced with culturally relevant ones in the target language to show a similar degree of effort.[26, 89]

CULTURAL VALIDITY

The degree to which the performance of the items on a translated or culturally adapted patient-reported outcome are an adequate reflection of the performance of items in the original version of the instrument. In the context of health assessment, translation of the words may not reflect the meaning in a different language or culture. Some wording or some concepts may not exist or be relevant in a different culture.[18]

D

DATA

Any organized information collected by a researcher; "data" is the plural term, the singular is "datum", but usage is quite inconsistent. Data are often thought of as statistical or quantitative, but they may take many other forms as well – such as transcripts of interviews or videotapes of social interactions. Non-quantitative data such as transcripts or videotapes are often coded or translated into numbers to make them easier to analyze.[90]

DATA SATURATION

A criterion to judge data adequacy in qualitative research operationalized as collecting data until no new information is obtained.[91]

DEBRIEFING

A process to carefully review a mission or an experience upon completion.[92]

DECISION AIDS

Interventions designed to help people make specific and deliberative choices among options by providing (at the minimum) information on the options and outcomes relevant to the person's health status. Additional strategies may include information on the disease or condition, probabilities of outcomes tailored to a person's health risk factors, an explicit values—clarification exercise, information on others' opinions, and guidance or coaching in the steps of decision-making and communicating with others. Decision aids may be administered with the use of various media, such as decision boards, interactive videodiscs, personal computers, audiotapes, audio-guided workbooks, pamphlets, and group presentations. Excluded from the definition of decision aids are: passive informed consent materials, educational interventions that are not geared to a specific decision, or interventions designed to promote compliance with a recommended option rather than a choice based on personal values.[93] Decision aids are needed when medical decisions are complex because of uncertain outcomes or the options have different risk-benefit profiles that patients value differently. Practice guidelines for these difficult decisions recommend that patients understand the probable outcomes of options; consider the personal value they place on benefits versus risks; and participate with their practitioners in deciding about treatment. Decision aids can be used as tools for shared decision making and as adjuncts to counselling from practitioners.[94]

DECISION ANALYSIS

The application of explicit, quantitative methods that quantify prognoses, treatment effects, and patient values in order to analyze a decision under conditions of uncertainty.[76]

DECISION-RELATED REGRET

A negative emotion associated with thinking about a past or future choice. The thinking component generally takes the form of a wish that things were otherwise and involves a comparison of what actually did or will take place with some better alternative—a "counterfactual thought." For predecisional (anticipated) regret, the thinking involves a mental simulation of the outcomes that might result from different choice options.[95] Decisional regret (also called decisional conflict) is a construct that can be measured[96] and decision aids are tools developed to help people make treatment decisions and avoid decisional regret. See also DECISION AIDS

DELPHI METHOD

A consensus building method, originally developed by the RAND Corporation in the 1950s to forecast the impact of technology on warfare. The method entails a group of experts who anonymously reply to questionnaires and subsequently receive feedback in the form of a statistical representation of the 'group response,' after which the process repeats itself. The goal is to reduce the range of responses and arrive at something closer to expert consensus. The Delphi Method has been widely adopted and is still in use today.[97-100]

DIFFERENTIAL ITEM FUNCTIONING (DIF)

A feature of test items such that they function differently for different groups of people, such as those defined by ethnic or socioeconomic status, as a result of DIF individuals with the same value of the latent variable having different probabilities of response depending on which group they belong to.[90]

DIRECT COSTS

Resources directly consumed by a program; direct health care costs include the cost of tests, drugs, supplies, health care personnel, and medical facilities.[87]

DISABILITY

Umbrella term for impairments, activity limitations or participation restrictions; negative aspects of functioning; terminology from the WHO's ICF framework.[7]

DISABILITY ADJUSTED LIFE YEARS

A measure of the burden of disease on a defined population and the effectiveness of interventions. They are based on adjustment of life expectancy to allow for long-term disability as estimated from official statistics. DALYs are calculated using a "disability weight" (a proportion less than 1) multiplied by chronologic age to reflect the burden of the disability. DALYs can thus produce estimates that accord greater value to fit than to disabled persons, and to the middle years of life rather than to youth or old age.[65]

DISABILITY PARADOX

Individuals with severe disabilities or limitations report having a good quality of life despite the fact that those without the disability or limitation think these individuals do not have a good quality of life. The concept of response shift is suggested as a mechanism explaining the "paradoxical and counter-intuitive" discrepancies between reported quality of life and 'expected quality of life'. However, others argue that the observation of high quality of life among people with disabilities is only 'paradoxical and counterintuitive' under the assumption that people with severe illness or disability have a poor quality of life by virtue of their illness or disability and this is the result of misperception and stereotypically negative attitudes on the part of people without disabilities. The implications of the disability paradox is that the 'counter intuitive discrepancies' that response shift seeks to explain may need to be more carefully, and independently, characterized as measurement issues.[101-103]

DISCORDANT

Term used in twin studies to describe a twin pair in which one twin exhibits a certain trait and the other does not; also used in matched pairs case-control studies to describe a pair whose members have different exposures to the risk factor under study. Only the discordant pairs are informative about the association between exposure and disease.[65]

DISCRETE CHOICE EXPERIMENT

Type of choice-based conjoint analysis in which patients' preferences for health states or health care scenarios are elicited by asking them to choose between selected pairs of scenarios (e.g. life expectancy of 12 years with severe problems with leaking urine versus life expectancy of 8 years with occasional problems with leaking urine). The main advantage of DCEs over the other methods of eliciting values such as standard gamble (SG) or time-trade-off (TTO) is that they allow the simultaneous assessment of multiple attributes rather than a dichotomous choice between one attribute and survival.[104]

DISCRIMINANT VALIDITY

A type of construct validity in which specific hypotheses are tested regarding how the measure under study relates to unrelated constructs as opposed to related constructs (convergent validity).[18]

DISEASE PREVENTION

The action of the health sector to deal with individuals and populations identified as exhibiting identifiable risk factors, often associated with different risk behaviours.[105]

DISEASE-SPECIFIC MEASURE

A health status instrument that is specific to a certain diagnosis or disease. Disease-specific measures are considered more responsive to change than generic measures.[106] Often wrongly used interchangeably with "condition-specific measure". See also CONDITION-SPECIFIC MEASURE.

DISMANTLING STUDY

A multi-component design or analysis that permits a disentangling of the different components of an effective intervention to determine which of the components/ingredients is responsible for the effect or outcome.[107]

DISSEMINATION

It is a planned process designed to facilitate research uptake in decision-making and practice involving the consideration of target audiences and the settings in which research findings are to be received and, where appropriate, communicating and interacting with wider policy and health service audiences. It involves identifying the appropriate audience and tailoring the message and medium to the audience. Dissemination activities can include such things as summaries, briefings to stakeholders, educational sessions with the public, patients, practitioners and/or policy makers, engaging knowledge users in developing and executing the dissemination or implementation plan, tools creation, and media engagement. It is a key element in the research-to-practice or knowledge translation continuum.[108, 109]

DISTRIBUTION-BASED

In the context of identifying change, this method relies on the statistical distributions of scores in a given study. These may include reliance on the standard deviation and/or standard error of measurement.[110] See also CHANGE.

DIVERGENT VALIDITY

See DISCRIMINANT VALIDITY.

DIVERSITY

The wide range of people's characteristics; age differences, race, gender, physical ability, sexual orientation, religion and language. Increasingly it also embraces background, professional experience, skills and specialisation, values and culture and social class.[12]

DOMAIN

In the context of measurement, it is a conceptually defined part of the construct; at the practical level, domains represent sub-scales of a measure with scores generated from the grouping of items related to that domain. The ICF defines a domain as a practical and meaningful set of related physiological functions, anatomical structures, actions, tasks, or areas of life. Under activity and participation category of the ICF, 9 domains are listed: learning and applying knowledge, general tasks and demands, communication, mobility, self-care, domestic life, interpersonal interactions and relationships, major life areas, community, social and civic life.[7]

DRUG SAFETY AND QUALITY

The safe, effective, appropriate, and efficient use of medications including the quality of the five components or subsystems of the medication use system; selecting and procuring the drug by the pharmacy, prescribing and selecting the drug for the patient, preparing and dispensing it, administering the drug, and monitoring the patient for effect. This does not include known risks associated with the medication itself, product purity, or integrity.[70]

DYAD

Two individuals maintaining a sociologically significant relationship. In the context of quality of life research, many health conditions affect "couples" as a unit when one member has to play a major caregiving or support role, resulting in reciprocal influence on many aspects of quality of life and well-being. Research in these areas needs to consider this dyadic phenomenon to fully appreciate their impact.[92, 111]

DYSFUNCTION

Impaired or abnormal functioning as of a body structure; abnormal or unhealthy interpersonal behavior or interaction within a group.[7]

E

E-HEALTH

E-health is the transfer of health resources and health care by electronic means. It encompasses three main areas: (1)The delivery of health information, for health professionals and health consumers, through the Internet and telecommunications; (2)Using the power of information technology (IT) and e-commerce to improve public health services, e.g. through the education and training of health workers; and (3)the use of e-commerce and e-business practices in health systems management.[34]

ECOLOGICAL FALLACY

Bias that may occur because an association observed between variables on an aggregate level does not necessarily represent the association that exists at an individual level. This type of bias can arise in health outcomes research for example if aggregate data, perhaps collected though a population level survey, on health perception or quality of life is linked another aggregate variable such as consumption of fruits and vegetables, hours of sunlight, or water quality, etc., and causal relationships are suggested. The fallacy is that this relationship may not hold when individual data on quality of life is linked statistically to individual data on consumption of fruits, vegetables, or water with different quality levels.[65, 112]

ECOLOGICAL PUBLIC HEALTH

A concept developed to respond to the changing nature of health issues arising from emerging global environmental deterioration (destruction of ozone layer, water and air pollution, and global warming). This concept emphasizes the common ground between achieving health and sustainable development and focuses on the economic and environmental determinants of health and the means by which economic investment should be guided towards producing the best population health outcomes greater equity in heath and sustainable use of resources.[105]

ECOLOGICAL VALIDITY

Degree to which results on a test or measure obtained in controlled experimental conditions are related to those obtained in real world environments. In health outcomes measurement, several examples come to mind such as neuropsychological testing or functional capacity testing on walking or dexterity tasks. Two approaches have been taken to address ecological validity of assessment instruments: verisimilitude and veridicality. Verisimilitude is the degree to which the demands (e.g. cognitive or motor) of a test theoretically resemble the demands in the everyday environment and usually requires developing new assessments that more closely simulate real world ability. Veridicality refers to the degree to which existing tests are empirically related to measures of everyday functioning and this would imply a statistical relationship between the test and real-world functioning. A test that demonstrates ecological validity is likely more predictive of how someone will function in daily life than a test that only has validity for diagnosis of impairment or measurement of severity.[113, 114]

EFFECT INDICATOR

See CAUSAL INDICATOR.

EFFECT MODIFICATION

Differing values of the effect measure at different levels of another variate, is an inherent characteristic of the relationship between two causes of an illness (effect). This relationship is not governed by the particulars of any study; it is an unalterable fact of nature.[42]

EFFECT SIZE

A general term for a statistical measure of the size of a relationship that is being investigated. There are many estimators (formulae) of effect size depending on the relationships being studied. For example, when two groups (such as a treatment group and a control group) are being compared and the outcome is measured on a continuous scale (value on an HRQL index), Cohen's effect size is the difference between groups/ standard deviation at baseline. Cohen's effect sizes have been categorized as trivial if <0.2, small for 0.2 to 0.5; medium for 0.5 to 0.8 and large for >0.8. In a correlational study, an effect size reflects the strength of the linear relationship between two variables and relationships are considered weak between 0.1 and 0.3, moderate if between 0.3 and 0.5 and strong if >0.5, however, the amount of variance explained (r^2) is not large unless r is >0.8. Studies of binary outcomes, effect sizes are expressed as odds ratios (OR) or relative risks (RR). Effect sizes are parameters and can be considered to have more clinical meaning than statistical probabilities. Effect sizes can be summarized across studies as is common using meta-analyses.[115-117]

EFFECTIVENESS

It is the measure of the extent to which a specific intervention, when deployed in the field under usual circumstances, does what it is intended to do for a specified population. This is distinguished from efficacy and efficiency.[5]

EFFICACY

The extent to which an intervention does more good than harm under ideal circumstances.[5]

EFFICIENCY

The extent to which the resources used to provide a specific intervention of known efficacy and effectiveness are minimized.[5]

EMOTIONAL SUPPORT

The availability of one or more persons who can listen sympathetically when an individual is having problems and can provide indications of caring and acceptance.[69]

EMOTIONAL VITALITY

A sense of positive energy, an ability to regulate behavior and emotions, and a feeling of engagement in life; this term has been used to characterize an individual's emotional response to adjusting to life with a chronic illness or injury and is considered to act as a critical buffer against the strain of living with a chronic illness or disability and enables some individuals to thrive and be emotionally vital in the process of recovery and adaptation. It comprises at least the five domains of (1) physical well-being and energy, (2) regulation of mood, (3) mastery, (4) engagement in meaningful roles and activities; and (5) feeling supported. In the context of positive psychology, the term resilience is often used, but in the context of rehabilitation, a construct parallel to physical vitality was desired to emphasize the need to address the "hidden disabilities", or the emotional aspects of managing functional loss.[118, 119]

EMOTIONAL WELL-BEING

One aspect of overall well-being, sometimes referred to as psychological well-being; other components include physical, functional, and social well being.[120, 121] See also WELL-BEING.

EMPOWERMENT

Social, cultural, psychological or political process through which individuals or social groups are able to express their needs, present their concerns, devise strategies for involvement in decision making, and achieve political, social and cultural action to meet those needs. Through the empowerment process, people see a closer correspondence between their goals in life and how to achieve them, and a relationship between their efforts and life outcomes.[105]

END-AVERSION BIAS

Refers to the reluctance of some people to use the extreme categories of a scale, often related to people's difficulty in making absolute judgements[4]; also called central tendency bias and is of particular feature of visual analogue scales.[4, 122]

ENDPOINT

In the context of the evaluation of an intervention, it is the outcome for which the efficacy or effectiveness will be judged; in an intervention trial, endpoints have been distinguished as primary, key secondary, or exploratory.[55]

ENVIRONMENTAL FACTOR

In the context of health, factors that make up the physical, social and attitudinal environment in which people live and conduct their lives.[7]

EPIDEMIOLOGY

The study of the distribution and determinants of health-states or events in specified populations, and the application of this study to the control of health problems.[65]

EQUITY

The absence of avoidable or remediable differences among populations or groups defined socially, economically, demographically, or geographically; thus, health inequities involve more than inequality—whether in health determinants or outcomes, or in access to the resources needed to improve and maintain health—but also a failure to avoid or overcome such inequality that infringes human rights norms or is otherwise unfair.[34]

EQUITY IN HEALTH

An assumption that people's needs guide the distribution of opportunities for well-being; it implies that all people have an equal opportunity to develop and maintain their health, through fair and just access to resources for health.[105]

ETHICALLY SOUND APPLICATION OF KNOWLEDGE

Ethically-sound knowledge translation activities for improved health are those that are consistent with ethical principles and norms, social values, as well as legal and other regulatory frameworks while keeping in mind that principles, values and laws can compete among and between each other at any given point in time. The term application is used to refer to the iterative process by which knowledge is put into practice.[108]

ETHNICITY

A sense of cultural and historical identity based on belonging by birth to a distinctive cultural group.[12]

ETHNOGRAPHY

A form of qualitative inquiry that is the process and product of describing and interpreting cultural behaviour; in this context, fieldwork, undertaken as participant observation, is the process by which to know a culture, and the product is written text portraying the culture which itself is not visible or tangible but is constructed by the act of ethnographic writing. It is a kind of phenomenology oriented towards describing the experience of everyday life as it is internalized in the subjective consciousness of individuals in an ongoing attempt to place specific encounters, events, and understandings into a fuller, more meaningful content.[38, 91]

EUDAIMONIA

A component of well-being comprising feelings of having purpose in life, personal growth, positive relations with others, environmental mastery, self-acceptance, and autonomy [123]

EVALUATION

The application of systematic methods to periodically and objectively assess effectiveness of programs in achieving expected results, their impacts (both intended and unintended), continued relevance and alternative or more cost-effective ways of achieving expected results.[124]

EVIDENCE

See HIERARCHY OF EVIDENCE.

EVIDENCE-BASED

Based on systematically reviewed clinical research findings.[52]

EVIDENCE-BASED MEDICINE

The conscientious, explicit and judicious use of current best evidence in making decisions about the care of individual patients.[76, 125]

EVIDENCE-BASED PRACTICE

The integration of (a) clinical expertise, (b) current best evidence, and (c) client values to provide high-quality services reflecting the interests, values, needs, and choices of the individuals served.[76]

EXACERBATIONS

These are clinical events characterized by a concerning change from the patient's previous status. Exacerbations are increasingly recognized as important outcomes to measure in clinical trials among diseases characterized by periodic functions in disease activity such as asthma, COPD, multiple sclerosis, and rheumatoid arthritis.[126] They can be quantified using annualized relapse rates.

EXCHANGE

The exchange of knowledge refers to the interaction between the knowledge user and the researcher, resulting in mutual learning. According to the Canadian Health Services Research Foundation (CHSRF), the definition of knowledge exchange is "collaborative problem-solving between researchers and decision makers that happens through linkage and exchange. Effective knowledge exchange involves interaction between knowledge users and researchers and results in mutual learning through the process of planning, producing, disseminating, and applying existing or new research in decision-making.[108]

EXERCISE

All planned, structured, repetitive and purposeful physical activities intended to improve or maintain physical fitness.[127, 128]

EXERCISE CAPACITY

Exercise capacity is the maximum amount of physical exertion that a person can sustain. An accurate assessment of exercise capacity requires that maximal exertion is sufficiently prolonged to have a stable (or *steady state*) effect on the circulation. During a graded exercise test, the gold standard for testing exercise capacity, the amount of oxygen required to generate the required work is measured. The parameter best representing exercise capacity is peak oxygen consumption (VO_2 peak)because most untrained test subjects never reach maximum oxygen consumption (VO_2

max). Exercise capacity is a more powerful predictor of mortality among men than other established risk factors for cardiovascular disease. It is also the target of all exercise interventions whether or not it is explicitly measured.[129-131]

EXISTENTIAL DISTRESS OR SUFFERING

In the context of palliative care, a concern about meaninglessness in present life, meaningless in past life, loss of social role functioning, feeling emotionally irrelevant, dependency, fear of being a burden on others, hopelessness, grief over imminent separation, "why me" questions, guilt, unfinished business, life after death, and faith.[132, 133]

EXPLANATORY HYPOTHESIS

In the context of a study on the efficacy or effectiveness of an intervention, some of the data collected would inform (explain) processes underlying achieving the outcome. Inclusion and testing of these explanatory hypotheses would not affect the power of the study to test the main effect (confirmatory hypothesis).[134]

EXPLORATORY FACTOR ANALYSIS

A statistical method that groups together those variables which are highly correlated with each other but are also relatively uncorrelated with other variables; these groups are then regarded as potential evidence of an underlying factor structure. Spearman first used EFA to explore aspects of intelligence[135] and it is widely used today as a form of construct validity in that if a measure comprises several different domains, then it should be possible to create clusters of items based on the item-to-item correlations; if the expected factors are produced, this contributes evidence for construct validity. EFA is a way of exploring data structure but it has been criticized as there may be many alternative and very different, factorizations possible and the factors may be difficult to interpret and/or inconsistent across studies.[40]

EXPLORATORY HYPOTHESIS

In the context of a study on the efficacy or effectiveness of an intervention, some of the data collected would inform the impact of the intervention on other outcomes that may be collateral or downstream from the main outcome. Inclusion and testing of these exploratory hypotheses would not affect the power of the study to test the main effect (confirmatory hypothesis).[134]

EXTERNAL VALIDITY

See GENERALIZABILITY.

EXTRAVERSION

Individual differences in the tendency to have a relatively positive view of the world and experience more positive affect. Extraverts are commonly described as bold, assertive, energetic and talkative. Extraversion has been shown to reliably predict alcohol consumption, popularity, parties attended, dating variety, and exercise.[136, 137]

F

FACE VALIDITY

The degree to which (the items of) an instrument indeed looks as though they are an adequate reflection of the construct to be measured.[46]

FACTOR ANALYSIS

A set of statistical methods for analyzing the correlations among several variables in order to estimate the number of fundamental dimensions that underlie the observed data and to describe and measure those dimensions. Used frequently in the development of scoring systems for rating scales and questionnaires.[65]

FACTOR LOADINGS

In structural equation modeling, the associations between latent variables and the observed measured variables are used to define them. They are interpreted as unstandardized regression coefficients estimating the effect of the latent factor on the indicator. The measured variable is the outcome variable, the latent variable is the explanatory variable, and the factor loading is the slope; factor loadings in standardized solutions are interpreted as correlations between the measured and latent variables, so long as the indicator loads on only a single factor. In the identification of response shift, a change in the pattern of factor loadings suggests reconceptualization. A change in the magnitude of factor loadings implies reprioritization.[50, 115]

FAMILY CAREGIVERS

Those individuals who are part of the immediate personal circle of a person with a health condition on whom s/he relies for support and care.[138]

FATIGUE

Is a clinically relevant symptom characterized by difficulty in initiation or sustaining voluntary activities and is distinguished from the lay notion of tiredness[139]. Perception of fatigue and performance fatigability are two components of fatigue which have different causes, manifestations and life impact.[140] There is no single agreed upon taxonomy for classifying fatigue. The following terms are used, albeit inconsistently, in the literature to refer to fatigue. The complexity of fatigue poses a challenge for measurement. See also SYMPTOM

1. PHYSIOLOGICAL FATIGUE (FATIGABILITY): Is the normal result of motor output and occurs if exercise continues to the point where muscle glycogen is depleted. It is commonly measured by physiological or performance tests on muscles.[128, 139] Physiological fatigue is only one component affecting initiation of or sustaining voluntary activities (work output) which is also influenced by cognitive and sensory factors, perceived exertion, motivation and incentives, and is also influenced by homeostatic (endocrine and autonomic) factors and the external environments (such as temperature).[139]

2. PATHOLOGICAL FATIGUE: An amplified sense of normal (physiological) fatigue that can be induced by changes in one or more variables regulating work output. In the presence of disease, fatigue could develop because of dissociation between the level of internal input (motivational and limbic) and the level of perceived exertion from the effort being into a task or activity. When there is loss of interest and motivation, as in depression, the subjective sense of fatigue is generated mainly as a result of reduced internal input.[139]

3. PERIPHERAL FATIGUE: Is muscle fatigability due to disorders of muscle and neuromuscular junction; often restored at least partially by rest.[128, 139]

4. CENTRAL FATIGUE: Often used synonymously with perception of fatigue, it is a feeling of constant exhaustion typically not improved by rest. Central fatigue is regulated by brain pathways associated with arousal and retention, reticular and limbic systems, and basal ganglia. Lesions in these pathways result in deterioration and fluctuation in severity of fatigue under physiological and psychological stimuli producing the perception of physical and perception of mental fatigue.

Mechanisms of central fatigue abnormalities in glucose metabolism and cerebral blood flow changes.[139]

5. MENTAL FATIGUE: is the cognitive component of central fatigue characterized by inability to sustain concentration and endure mental tasks. It is assessed by measuring deterioration in cognitive performance on tests of cognitive processing administered over time (typically several hours).[139]

6. CANCER RELATED FATIGUE: Is an unusual and ongoing tiredness occurring with cancer or cancer treatments; described as overwhelming, it interferes with everyday life and it is not always relieved by rest.[11]

7. CHRONIC FATIGUE: Is not a clinical entity except in the context of CHRONIC FATIGUE SYNDROME, which is defined as a disabling fatigue with a combination of symptoms that must be persistent or relapsing for 6 months or more and affecting activities of daily living. In addition to fatigue to be diagnosed with the syndrome people must report at least 4 of the following symptoms: impaired memory and/or concentration, sore throat, tender cervical and/or axillary lymph nodes, muscle pain, multi-joint pain, new headaches, unrefreshing sleep and post-exertional malaise[141-143].

8. MULTIPLE SCLEROSIS FATIGUE: Is a severe and frequent impediment to sustained physical functioning, often of sudden onset, slow to recover, precipitated or accentuated by heat and/or humidity, leading to a sustained or chronic state that is not always correlated with other MS symptoms.[144]

FEASIBILITY

In the context of research or clinical care, this refers to the question of whether or not study participants or patients are able to do something.[18]

FIDELITY

Adherence to prescribed treatment elements and to standards of competency or skill delivery. In the context of quality of life research, many of the interventions that directly target quality of life are difficult to apply consistently, even in the research setting, and can vary by practitioner, site, and time. In this context, measuring fidelity would be important way of identifying bias and/or variability.[145, 146]

FITNESS

See EXERCISE CAPACITY.

FIVE FACTOR MODEL OF PERSONALITY

Fundamental dimensions along which personality traits cluster across individuals: Extraversion, Agreeableness, Conscientiousness, Neuroticism, and Openness to Experience. The five factors have been shown to have convergent and discriminant validity across instruments and observers and to endure across decades in adults; consensus on the five factors took 20 years of study across disciplines, cultures, and countries, researchers.[147, 148]

FLOOR AND CEILING EFFECTS

Occur when a high proportion of the population scores at either the lower or upper end of the scale. This occurs when the items are either too hard or too easy for the sample being tested. These effects may impact on the capacity to detect change but the importance of floor and ceiling effects will depend on whether change in these groups is of interest. For example, the tests of physical capacity may be too hard for many people with health conditions and the vast majority will have values at the very low end. If there is no interest in detecting further deterioration in exercise capacity, the floor effect may not be a consequence. However, a scale that has a high ceiling effect because the items are too easy, a feature of many ADL measures, will have a large proportion of respondents scoring at the top end. Even if people improved no further positive change could be detected[2]. This is one of the reasons that the concept of instrumental activities of daily living was conceived to reflect problems more typically experienced by people with less severe forms of disability and who live freely in the community and need to shop, cook and manage money in addition to basic ADL.[149]

FLOW

State of heightened focus and immersion in activities such as art, play and work which is a state in which people are the happiest; flow is best achieved when there is a balance between the challenge of the task and the skill of the performer, the best match being achieved when the skill level and challenge measures are high, sometimes referred to as "being in the zone".[150]

FOCUS GROUP

Focus groups are a form of group interview that capitalises on communication between research participants in order to generate data; the interaction is used explicitly as part of the method.[151]

FORCED-CHOICE

Method to avoid *Yea-Saying* by having respondents choose between two choices rather than agreeing or disagreeing with a list of choices.[152]

FORMATIVE CONSTRUCT

See CONCEPTUAL MODEL.

FORWARD TRANSLATION

The process of translating a measure from the original language of development, the source language, into another language, the target language. This is one of several steps required to produce a valid translation. Translation involves a combination of the literal translation of individual words and sentences from one language to another and an adaptation with regard to idiomatic expressions, and to cultural context and lifestyle. Languages with similar structure, such as the European languages, require less adaptation, during translations but translation from a European language to Arabic or Asian languages would require more adaptation. The process of translation is rigorous and requires at least two independent translators, or even better, teams of translators. Qualified translators need to carry out the translation but highly educated individuals may not be culturally representative of the target population; translators should preferably translate into their mother tongue. Some of the translators should be aware of the objectives and concepts provide a more reliable representation of the material to be translated but other translators should be naive as they could offer a different insight into the translation.[26] See also TRANSLATABILITY ASSESSMENT, BACK TRANSLATION, CULTURAL ADAPTATION

FRAILTY

One of the health-related characteristics that are associated with increasing age along with disability, comorbidity; frailty is a result of health problems overwhelming the physiological, psychological, and social reserves of an older person leaving them vulnerable to functional decline.[153, 154]

FRAME OF REFERENCE

A set of experiences from the physical, mental or environmental contexts used by a person to anchor a response to a question about a health or quality of life state. Examples are past state, states of others, and expectations. Over time, the frame of reference to anchor a response may change and this change is a factor contributing to response shift.[24]

FUNCTION

Umbrella term encompassing all body functions, activities and participation; positive aspects of disability; terminology from the World Health Organization's ICF framework.[7]

G

GAMMA

Gamma coefficient is a measure of the relationship between two ordinal variables, however, the assumption of presumed normal is not a requirement and the value is not very much affected by outliers. It is applied to estimate the extent of agreement on two ranked variables usually with relatively few categories and many ties.[155]

GENDER

The cultural meanings ascribed to male and female social categories.[156]

GENDER IDENTITY

Masculine and feminine self-definitions in terms of the culturally typical or ideal man or woman; one's psychological relationship to male and female social categories.[156]

GENDER PERSPECTIVE

Way of looking at situations and issues taking into account the respective roles and contributions of men and women in society.[156]

GENDER ROLES

The array of socially constructed roles and relationships, personality traits and attitudes, behaviors, values, relative power and influence that society ascribes to two sexes based on a differential basis. These roles are manifested by the interrelationship between men and women in the context of their society and roles in that society and are the patterns of behaviour, rights and obligations defined by a society as appropriate for each sex. Gender roles and characteristics do not exist in isolation, but are defined in relation to one another.[156]

GENERAL HEALTH PERCEPTION

See HEALTH PERCEPTION.

GENERALIZABILITY

The ability to generalize study findings beyond the target population to all members of the population or people with the health condition of interest; also sometimes termed external validity. A common challenge in research is to achieve a balance between bias (internal validity) and generalizability. Randomized clinical trials are designs that typically focus on reducing bias and may, as a consequence, have limited generalizability.[17]

GRIEF

An unhappy and painful emotion occurring as a reaction to a major loss. Grief may be triggered by the death of a loved one, or if they have an illness for which there is no cure, or a chronic condition that affects their quality of life. The end of a significant relationship may also cause a grieving process. Five stages of grief have been recognized: denial, anger, bargaining, depressed mood, acceptance. These reactions might not occur in a specific order, and can (at times) occur together. Not everyone experiences all of these emotions.[30]

GROUNDED THEORY

An approach aimed at developing theories, concepts, or models beginning from the data. Grounded theory methodology uses a set of specific and rigorous procedures for producing substantive theory of social phenomena using techniques of induction, deduction, and verification; methodology involves an iterative process involving experience with the data to generate hypotheses or insights which are pursued with further data collection employing a method termed constant comparison.[38]

GUTTMAN SCALING

Multiple items measuring a uni-dimensional construct in which the items are chosen to have a hierarchical order of difficulty.[18]

H

HANDICAP

Older terminology that refers to restrictions that a person has in participating in life's roles; in the WHO's ICF model. "Handicap" is the situational result of an interaction between a person's profile of disabilities arising from disease or trauma and environmental characteristics that may have created a sociocultural or physical obstacles to participate or engage in family life roles and/or opportunities for employment, education, recreation, or economic self-sufficiency.[7, 157]

HAPPINESS

Aristotle's definition of eudaimonia as the highest of all goods achievable by human action[158] is considered to mean happiness. This eudaimonic view is that the good life is achieved by maximizing potential rather than solely pursuing pleasure (hedonism).[159] In psychology, happiness is operationalized as achieving a balance between positive and negative affect.[160] The English word "happiness" dates to the 14th century from the word "hap" meaning fortune or chance. While hap is no longer used, hapless survives and means unfortunate. To be happy was at first considered to be favoured by fortune but in the 16th century it came to mean pleasure.[161] Happiness has been a constant theme and embedded in the American constitution, but as Benjamin Franklin (1706-1709), Founding Father of the United States, pointed out, *"The constitution only guarantees the American people the right to pursue happiness. You have to catch it yourself."* The English writer and politician, Joseph Addison (1672-1719), made a suggestion as to how to make this catch reminiscing that, *"Three grand essentials to happiness in this life are something to do, something to love, and something to hope for."* Happiness is a constant topic in popular culture, immortalized through song and film, and several definitions have been proposed. *"Happiness is a warm gun"*, a 1968 Beatles song released on the White Album and written by John Lennon, defines happiness as a drug fix. In the 1966 song by WH Weatherspoon "What Becomes of the Broken-

Hearted?", "*happiness is an illusion, filled with sadness and confusion*". In the 1967 musical, the Peanuts character, Charlie Brown, defines happiness as "*anyone and anything at all that's loved by you*". In the 2014 movie, Despicable Me 2, Pharrell Williams encourages "*Clap along if you feel like happiness is the truth*" and "*Clap along if you know what happiness is to you*". Perhaps more illuminating is that one of the conclusion from the 2011 documentary "Happy" (Wadi Films Inc.), is that happiness is 50% genetics, 10% circumstance (hap), and 40% actions a person does intentionally to derive happiness such as those related to personal growth, fostering close connected relationships, and making the world a better place (both hedonistic and eudaimonic actions).

Happiness, like many other important constructs related to well-being is culturally specific. In Western societies, it is defined mostly in terms of eudaimonia and hedonism; in Eastern societies, it is defined more in terms of what high state of being can be achieved in the future. The popular western view includes the concept of being loved and loving. In sum, happiness is recognition of a positive state of well-being derived from doing good, from finding pleasure in current circumstances and loving relationships, and from hope. You can't have happiness without knowing it and happiness can be transient depending on "hap".

The former would be considered a definition of happiness from an individual perspective. From a global perspective, the 2015 World Happiness Report[162], identified six factors reflecting happiness from a country perspective: Gross Domestic Product (GDP) per capita, healthy years of life expectancy, social support (as measured by having someone to count on in times of trouble), trust (as measured by a perceived absence of corruption in government and business), perceived freedom to make life decisions, and generosity (as measured by recent donations, adjusted for differences in income). Based on this definition, the five happiest countries in 2015 were Switzerland, Iceland, Denmark, Norway, and Canada.

HAZARD/ HAZARD RATIO

See COX'S PROPORTIONAL HAZARD RATIO.

HEALTH

A state of complete physical, social and mental well-being, and not merely the absence of disease or infirmity. Health is a fundamental human right and is considered a resource for everyday life, and not the object of living. It is a positive concept emphasizing social and personal resources as well as physical capabilities. The prerequisites for health include peace, adequate economic resources, food and shelter, and a stable ecosystem and sustainable resources use.[105, 163]

HEALTH BEHAVIOR

Any activity undertaken by an individual for the purpose of promoting, protecting or maintaining health, whether or not such behavior is objectively effective toward that end.[163]

HEALTH EDUCATION

Consciously constructed opportunities for learning to improve health literacy, knowledge and life skills conducive to individual health and healthy communities. Health education not only provides opportunities to communicate information but also to foster the motivation, skills and confidence (self-efficacy) necessary to take action to improve health.[105]

HEALTH EXPECTANCY

A population-based measure of the proportion of expected life span estimated to be healthful and fulfilling, or free of illness, disease and disability, according to social norms and perceptions and professional standards. Health expectancy indicators quantify the extent to which individuals experience a life span free of disability, disorders, and/or chronic disease. Two indicators are disability free life years (DFLY) and quality adjusted life years (QALY).[32]

HEALTH IMPACT ASSESSMENT (HIA)

A multidisciplinary process within which a range of evidence about the health effects of a proposal is considered in a structured framework. It is based on a broad model of health which proposes that economic, political, social, psychological, and environmental factors determine population health. HIAs are used to document the long-term health effects of investments, policies and projects in other sectors that affect social and physical environments. Examples include projects in community design, transportation planning, and other areas outside the traditional realm of public health concerns. HIAs serve to: make the health and equity impacts of social decisions more explicit; provide an accountability mechanism to prevent harm; shape projects, plans, and policies to promote and improve the population's health, and support meaningful, inclusive participation in governance institutions.[164]

HEALTH INDICATOR

A characteristic of an individual, population, or environment which is subject to measurement (directly or indirectly) and can be used to describe one or more aspects of the health of an individual or population in terms of quality, quantity and time.[32]

HEALTH INEQUITIES

Avoidable inequalities in health between groups of people within countries and between countries; they are considered avoidable because they arise from inequalities within and between societies rather than from biological differences. Social and economic conditions and their effects on people's lives determine their risk of illness; they also determine actions taken to prevent and treat illness; also termed health disparities.[165]

HEALTH LITERACY

Degree to which individuals have the capacity to obtain, process, and understand basic health information and services needed to make appropriate health decisions; as such it represents the cognitive and social skills which determine the motivation and ability of individuals to gain access to, understand and use information in ways which promote and maintain good health.[7, 105, 166-168]

HEALTH OUTCOME

An aspect of an individual's physical, emotional, mental or social health that is expected to change owing to a deliberate intervention or to vary in the presence of another personal, health or environmental factor.[169]

HEALTH PERCEPTION

A construct that represents how individuals integrate objective information they have about their health with how they feel about or evaluate that information; this construct covers perceptions of both physical and mental health status along with other health related perception such as worry and concern about health perceived resistance or susceptibility to illness and sickness orientation with the tendency to believe that illness is a part of life. This is an important construct because the majority of physician office visits are initiated by patients because of how they feel.[170, 171]

HEALTH PROMOTION

The process of enabling people to increase control over the determinants of health and thereby improve their health. It represents a comprehensive social and political process embracing actions for strengthening skills and capabilities of individuals, but also actions directed towards changing social, environmental and economic conditions. Health promotion requires three strategies: (i) advocacy to create the essential conditions for health; (ii) enabling all people to achieve their full health potential, and (iii) mediating between the different interests in society in the pursuit of health.[105, 163]

HEALTH PROMOTING HOSPITAL

A hospital that provides not only high quality comprehensive medical and nursing services, but also develops a corporate identity that embraces the aims of health promotion. Such hospitals take action to promote the health of their patients, their staff, and the population within the community they are located.[172]

HEALTH RELATED QUALITY OF LIFE (HRQL)

A term referring to the health aspects of quality of life, generally considered to reflect the impact of disease and treatment on disability and daily functioning; it has also been considered to reflect the impact of perceived health on an individual's ability to live a fulfilling life. However, most specifically HRQL is a measure of the value assigned to duration of life as modified by impairments, functional states, perceptions and opportunities, as influenced by disease, injury, treatment and policy.[173]

HEALTH RELATED QUALITY OF LIFE IN ANIMALS (HRQL-A)

There is no reason why the concept of HRQL should apply only to people as animals suffer many of the same symptoms and activity limitations that impact on HRQL as do people. Animals can't speak for themselves but do have observable affective responses to their circumstances and their owners can report on these responses. The observable features that owners can report on are changes in behaviour, attitude, and demeanour. The following domains have been identified as pertaining to HRQL in dogs: activity, comfort, appetite, extroversion-introversion, aggression, anxiety, alertness, dependence, contentment, consistency, agitation, posture-mobility and compulsion.[174-179] See also QUALITY OF LIFE IN ANIMALS

HEALTH SERVICES RESEARCH

A field of inquiry that examines the impact of the organization, financing and management of health care services on the delivery, quality, cost, access to and outcomes of such services.[34]

HEALTH STATE

The health of an individual at any particular point in time. A health state may be modified by the impairments, functional states, perceptions, and social opportunities that are influenced by disease, injury, treatment, or health policy.[180]

HEALTH STATE CLASSIFICATION SYSTEM

An approach used to identify and label dimensions and their levels of functioning to describe general and specific health states.[181]

HEALTH STATUS

Description and/or measurement of the health of an individual or population at a particular point in time against identifiable standards.[34]

HEALTH TARGET

The amount of change in a specific measurable health outcome or intermediate health outcome that could reasonably be expected for a defined population within a defined time period. As such health targets define the concrete steps which may be taken to achieve a healthy goal.[105]

HIERARCHY OF EVIDENCE

In the context of evidence-based practice, this refers to the ranking of the strength of evidence for treatment benefits. Note that the absence of evidence is not the same as evidence against a health intervention.

1 (a) Meta-analysis of RCTs

1 (b) Individual high quality RCT with narrow confidence intervals

2 (a) Meta-analysis of cohort studies

2 (b) Individual cohort study (including low quality RCT; e.g. <80% follow-up)

3 (a) Meta-analysis of case-control studies

3 (b) Individual Case-Control Study

4 Case series (and poor quality cohort and case-control studies)

5 Expert opinions without explicit critical appraisal, or based on physiology, bench research or "first principles"

6. No evidence yet [76]

HOT DECK

A method of replacing missing data using a subset of the population that closely matches the individuals with the missing data. The name comes from the era when punch cards were used for computing. The operator set the criteria for selecting the matching sample. When the cards were selected from the card sorter, they were warm and hence the name hot deck.[66]

I

IGNORABLE MISSING DATA

See MISSING DATA.

IMPAIRMENT

Problems in body function or structure such as a significant deviation or loss.[7]

IMPLICIT THEORY OF CHANGE (ITC)

An explanation of how people consider the extent to which they have changed on some aspect of health over a fixed time period. This theory is based on the premise that people cannot accurately recall the initial state, compare it to their current state, and carry out some mental calculation, but rather, use some experience-based techniques to arrive at an estimate of change. This estimate may not be optimal but considered "good enough" for the situation. The judgment of change under ITC is based on a process that begins with the current state and works backwards considering how much things have changed over the time period. Therefore ITC is a process whereby people estimate the extent of change over a fixed time by considering time course of change rather than an analysis based on health states at specific times. ITC differs from her response shift recalibration where, using the then test, people are asked to re-rate a past rating based on current experience. Using an ITC lens and recognizing that people want to improve, especially from health conditions that require considerable effort to achieve gains, the re-rating carried out using the then test would likely be biased (usually lower), whereas the change value using ITC would be more accurate.[182]

IMPUTATION

The practice of 'filling in' missing data with plausible values is an attractive approach to analyzing incomplete data. It apparently solves the missing-data problem at the beginning of the analysis. However, a naive or unprincipled imputation method may create more problems than it solves, distorting estimates, standard errors and hypothesis tests.[183] See also MULTIPLE IMPUTATION.

INCEPTION COHORT

See COHORT STUDY

INCIDENCE

The number of new cases of a disease that occur during a specified period of time in a population at risk for developing the disease.[17]

INCREMENTAL COSTS

The difference in cost or effect between two or more programs being compared.[87]

INDEX

A psychometrically sound collection of items with an underlying theoretical framework that distinguishes between interrelated constructs relevant to a given health condition. The index may consist of multiple items that are aggregated into collective scores, representing component constructs or aspects of a condition. It may also be simply a single item.[51]

INDICATOR VARIABLE

In the context of the assessment of a latent construct, these are variables that reflect a level of ability or state of mind but they do not alter or influence the latent construct that they measure; as an example, many items reflect anxiety/depression but these items do not necessarily cause depression/anxiety.[41]

INDIRECT COSTS

A term used to refer to productivity losses. Time is a common component of indirect costs.[87]

INDIVIDUALIZED (quality of life) MEASURES

Measures of quality of life designed to capture the true meaning of quality of life, essentially defining quality of life as what the individual determines it to be, by allowing the patient to identify the domains (or areas of life) that are important to them, and to assign a weight on the relative importance of each one.[184, 185]

INDIVIDUALIZED MEDICINE

See PERSONALIZED MEDICINE.

INFORMATIONAL SUPPORT

Providing knowledge that is useful for solving problems, such as providing advice and guidance about alternative courses of action.[69]

INFORMED CONSENT

Refers to the requirement that all researchers explain the purposes, risks, benefits, confidentiality protections, and other relevant aspects of a research study to potential humans[19] and that all persons who participate in research should do so voluntarily, understanding the purpose of the research, and its risks and potential benefits, as fully as reasonably possible.[186]

INSTITUTE OF MEDICINE

Established in 1970, the IOM is the health arm of the National Academy of Sciences, which was chartered under President Abraham Lincoln in 1863. It is an independent, non-profit organization that works outside of government to provide unbiased and authoritative advice to decision makers and the public. The IOM asks and answers the nation's most pressing questions about health and health care. The aim is to help those in government and the private sector make informed health decisions by providing evidence upon which they can rely.[70]

INSTRUMENT (TOOL)

Terms used to describe a measuring device which could be a collection of self-report items or a physical device. It is best used to describe a physical device.[51]

INSTRUMENTAL ACTIVITIES OF DAILY LIVING (IADL)

Activities with aspects of cognitive and social functioning, including shopping, cooking, doing housework, managing money and using the telephone.[187]

INSTRUMENTAL SUPPORT

Involves practical help when necessary, such as assisting with transportation, helping with household chores and childcare, and providing tangible aid such as bringing tools or lending money.[69]

INTANGIBLE COSTS

Term used to describe consequences that are difficult to measure including costs of pain, suffering, grief, and other nonfinancial outcomes.[87]

INTEGRATED CARE

A coherent set of methods and models in the funding, administrative, organisational, service delivery and clinical levels designed to create connectivity, alignment and collaboration within and between the cure and care sectors. Integration is of services related to diagnosis, treatment care, rehabilitation and health promotion with the aim of improving access, quality, user satisfaction and efficiency.[188, 189]

INTEGRATED CARE PATHWAY

A tool and a concept that embeds guidelines, protocols and locally agreed, evidence-based, person-centred, best practices into everyday use for the individual.[12]

INTENTION-TO-TREAT (ITT)

In the context of an RCT, it is an analytical framework in which all randomized subjects are analyzed according to original treatment assignment, and all events are counted against the assigned treatment. ITT permits the testing of the policy of offering treatment and considers that the treatment is provided in a context and that it will not always be delivered as recommended—or at all. Provision for departures from protocol and other problems is a critical part of the policy, and this is the reason for intention-to-treat analysis.[190, 191]

INTER-RATER RELIABILITY

The extent to which two or more raters, independently rating a stable group of people under the identical conditions, agree on the score.[65]

INTERMEDIATE HEALTH OUTCOME

Changes in the determinants of health (lifestyles and living conditions) attributable to a planned intervention or interventions.[105]

INTERMEDIATE VARIABLE

A variable that acts in the causal pathway from an exposure or independent variable to an outcome (dependent variable). It causes the exposure variable to act upon the outcome. Adjusting for such a variable in a regression model would result in removing the effect of the exposure variable. Also called a contingent, intervening, or mediator variable).[65]

INTERNAL CONSISTENCY

See CRONBACH'S ALPHA.

INTERNATIONAL CLASSIFICATION, FUNCTIONING, DISABILITY, AND HEALTH (ICF)

A unified and standard language and framework for the description of health and health-related states. It defines components of well-being (such as education and labour). The domains contained in the ICF can, therefore, be seen as health domains and health-related domains. These domains are described from the perspective of the body, the individual and society in two basic lists: (1) Body Functions and Structures; and (2) Activities and Participation. As a classification, ICF systematically groups different domains for a person in a given health condition (e.g. what a person with a disease or disorder does do or can do).[7]

INTERPRETABILITY

The degree to which one can assign qualitative meaning—that is, clinical or commonly understood connotations to an instrument's quantitative scores or change in scores.[46]

INTERVAL SCALE

See MEASUREMENT SCALE.

INTRACLASS CORRELATION COEFFICIENT

Intraclass correlation (ICC) is used to measure inter-rater reliability for two or more raters. It may also be used to assess test-retest reliability. ICC may be conceptualized as the ratio of between-groups variance to total variance.[18]

INTRA-RATER CONSISTENCY

This is a type of reliability assessment in which the same assessment is completed by the same rater on two or more occasions. These different ratings are then compared, generally by means of correlation; as the same individual is completing both assessments, the rater's subsequent ratings are contaminated by knowledge of earlier ratings.[18]

ITEM

A single question that can stand alone or be part of a series of loosely affiliated questions or part of a psychometrically sound measurement index. [51]

ITEM RESPONSE THEORY (IRT)

A statistical theory and set of mathematical models expressing the probability of a particular response to a scale item as a function of the quantitative (latent) attribute of the person and of certain characteristics (parameters) of the item with the aim of precisely estimating a person's value on the latent trait based on responses to a series of categorical variables. Two key assumptions of IRT models are: (i) unidimensionality meaning only one latent trait is measured by the items; and (ii) local or conditional independence, meaning that there is no relationship between a person's responses to different items in the scale once the person's level on the latent trait into account. Different mathematical models apply depending on whether the responses are binary or polytomous. The three most popular unidimensional dichotomous (binary) IRT models are the one-, two-,and three-parameter logistic (PL) models whose names are associated with the number of item parameters that characterize an item's functioning and, thus, need to be estimated. The one-parameter logistic model (1PLM) estimates only item difficulty similar to models belonging to the family of Rasch models. The two-parameter model (2PLM) estimates difficulty and discrimination among people which varies across items. The three parameter model (3PLM) estimates difficulty, discrimination and guessing, although guessing is not usually a feature of responding to questions on health outcomes and, hence, the 3PLM has not been found to add any information for health outcomes measurement. For polytomous responses the most common models are Partial Credit Model, Rating Scale Model, Generalized Partial Credit Model, Graded Response Model, and Nominal Response Model the application of which depend on the assumptions about discrimination power across items, ordering responses, and distance between the item thresholds.[192-195] See also RASCH ANALYSIS

J

JACKKNIFE

A statistical procedure for reducing bias in estimation and providing approximate confidence intervals for parameters where these cannot be obtained in the usual way. The procedure involves removing from the sample each person in turn, yielding n samples of size n-1. This process yields n estimates of the parameter of interest which can be used to derive a more realistic estimate of the parameter and an estimate of standard error.[3]

K

KAPLAN-MEIER ESTIMATE

A non parametric method for creating a life or survival table by combining calculated probabilities of survival and withdrawal or censoring at each time an event occurs (outcome or withdrawal); censoring is assumed to occur at random and time intervals for calculation of probabilities are unequal because they are determined by the timing of events.[65]

KAPPA

A measure of the degree of non-random agreement between observers (raters) or measurements of the same categorical variable; sometimes referred to as chance corrected agreement; it is calculated as the ratio of (observed agreement – expected agreement) to (1 – expected agreement). There are different formulations of kappa depending on the number of categories of classification, two (Cohen's kappa) or more than two (Fleiss's kappa). For more than two categories, weighted kappa is calculated with weights depending upon the seriousness of the disagreement such as off by one category or off by more than one. Several magnitude guidelines have been suggested but none are universally accepted. Landis and Koch characterized values as: <0 as indicating no agreement; 0–0.20 as slight, 0.21–0.40 as fair, 0.41–0.60 as moderate, 0.61–0.80 as substantial, and 0.81–1 as almost perfect agreement. Fleiss characterized kappas over 0.75 as excellent, 0.40 to 0.75 as fair to good, and below 0.40 as poor. Kappa has some paradoxical values based on situations where expected agreement is very high as when the prevalence of one category is very high. When reporting kappa, reporting also crude or observed agreement and expected agreement helps in the interpretation of the value of kappa.[5, 16, 196]

KNOWLEDGE TRANSLATION (KT)

A dynamic and iterative process that includes synthesis, dissemination, exchange, and ethically sound application of knowledge to improve the health of individuals, provide more effective health services and products and strengthen the health care system. This process takes place within a complex system of interactions between researchers and knowledge users, which may vary in intensity, complexity and level of engagement depending on the nature of the research and the findings as well as the needs of the particular knowledge user. The evaluation and monitoring of KT initiatives, processes, and activities are key components of the KT process.[108, 197]

KNOWN GROUPS METHOD

A typical method to support construct validity and is based on forming hypotheses about how a measure undergoing validation behaves when comparing between a group of individuals known to have a particular trait and a group who do not have the trait; may also be used for hypotheses about individuals with differing levels/severities of a trait. The known groups methods will evaluate the test's ability to discriminate between the groups based on the groups demonstrating different mean scores on the test.[198] In a classic known-groups validation study, Weissman et al. compared Center for Epidemiologic Studies-Depression (CES-D) scores between groups of patients diagnosed with depression to a community-based sample. The large differences in CES-D scores between groups and the pattern of differences supported the construct validity of the CES-D. Known groups may be studied using groups of individuals with differing levels or severities of a characteristic.[199, 200] See also MINIMAL IMPORTANT DIFFERENCE (MID)

L

LATE EFFECTS

Side effects of cancer treatment that appear months or years after treatment has ended. Late effects include physical and mental problems and second cancers.[52]

LATENT CONSTRUCTS

Latent constructs are not directly observable or quantifiable.[201]

LATENT VARIABLE

1. Also known as a latent factor.[202]
2. There have been many definitions[203] of latent variables (also known as a latent factor) largely due to different statistical models including:
   a. Hypothethical variables that scientists put together out of their imaginations[88];
   b. A construct that cannot be seen or directly measured, such as 'happiness' or 'quality of life'.
   c. Unobservable or unmeasurable constructs, implying now and in the future;
   d. Variables that create an association between observed variables such that if the latent variables are held constant, the observed variables are independent (local independence definition);
   e. The true score that would be obtained if replicated responses could be obtained independently;
   f. A variable in a linear structural equation system that cannot be expressed as a function of manifest or measured variables; in this statistical method, latent variables are designated with an oval, and are associated with measured variables which are affected by the latent variable.
   g. A variable for which there is no sample realization for at least some observations in a given sample, implying that all variables are latent until sample values of them are available

(this is the only definition that is not model dependent). Latent variables can be derived from the data (a posterior) or hypothesized prior to examination of the data (a priori).[88, 203]

LEISURE

Activity that promotes the refreshment of health or spirits by relaxation and enjoyment; it goes beyond just time not working or doing other duties, as the time is for personal pleasure.[12]

LEVELS OF EVIDENCE

See HIERARCHY OF EVIDENCE.

LIFE HISTORY METHODOLOGY

A variety of qualitative approaches that focuses on the generation, analysis, and presentation of the data of a life history and the unfolding of an individual's experiences over time; it takes the view that human action can best be understood from the accounts and perspective of people involved and, thus, the focus is on an individual's subjective definition and experience of life.[38]

LIFE SKILLS

Personal, interpersonal, cognitive and physical skills which enable people to control and direct their lives, and to develop the capacity to live with and produce change in their environment.   Skills in decision-making, problem-solving, creative and critical thinking, self-awareness, communication, coping with emotions, and managing stress are key life skills that are the building blocks to the development of personal skills for health promotion.[105]

LIFE-SPACE MOBILITY

A spatial measure of the area through which a person travels over a specified time period ranging from displacement extending from within one's own home to displacement beyond one's town or geographic region. It has been shown to correlate well with diary records of daily activities over a one month period and is highly correlated with performance measures such as gait speed and balance.[204, 205]   It could serve as an indicator of participation as defined by the ICF. See also INTERNATIONAL CLASSIFICATION, FUNCTIONING, DISABILITY, AND HEALTH (ICF)

LIKERT ITEM and LIKERT SCALE

A Likert item is a response format consisting of options for indicating degree of agreement with a proposed statement; Likert items commonly have 5 to 7 options, and the inclusion of a neutral mid-point is optional. A Likert scale is a multi-item scale commonly used for measuring attitudes or beliefs. The following sample item from the Satisfaction with Life Scale by Diener et al. 1985 illustrates use of a 7-point Likert item: I am satisfied with my life. 1= strongly disagree/2=disagree/4= slightly disagree/5= neither agree nor disagree/6=agree/7=strongly agree.[206-208]

LIST WISE DELETION

A method of dealing with missing data, that is usually the default option in statistical packages, whereby any cases (people in the study) with missing data are excluded from the analysis; this can seriously reduce the sample size for analysis if there are many variables with even a small proportion of missing on any one variable; also called case wise deletion or complete case analysis.[66] This approach to analysis should be avoided.

LONGITUDINAL STUDY

See PROSPECTIVE COHORT STUDY.

LONGITUDINAL VALIDITY

Validity of change scores as indicated by the extent to which changes on one measure correlate with changes on another measure.[2]

M

MANIFEST VARIABLE

In the context of the assessment of a latent construct, these are the observed responses made by respondents to the questionnaire items.[41]

MANN WHITNEY U TEST

The Mann Whitney U test is a nonparametric test that compares two independent samples; it is more efficient (needs less sample size to identify an effect) than the t-test when the distributions are not normal. The test is based on ranking each subject ignoring group and then calculating the sum of the ranks of the separate groups and comparing these using the U statistic.[209]

MARGIN

The costs of producing one extra unit of output.[87]

MARKER

A diagnostic indication that disease may develop.[52]

MEASURE

A term often used to describe a questionnaire, index, checklist, instrument, or tool when in the context of modern measurement theory it should only be used as a verb (as to measure) or to describe a set of items that have been shown to form a unidimensional linear continuum.

MEASUREMENT

Rules for assigning symbols to objects in order to numerically represent quantities of attributes and includes evaluating numbers such that they reflect the differing degrees of the attribute being measured.[88]

MEASUREMENT ERROR

The systematic and random error of a value on a test or measure that is not attributed to true changes in the construct to be measured.[46]

MEASUREMENT SCALE

The range of possible values for a measurement (e.g., the set of possible responses to a question, the physically possible range for a set of biophysical measurements). Measurement scales that can only take certain values are labelled discrete or categorical; scales that can take on any value depending on the precision of the measuring device are continuous. The measurement scale can be inherent to the construct or created for statistical or interpretability purposes. See also CORRELATION. Measurement scales can be further classified according to the quantitative character of the scale; the choice of statistical analysis depends on the measurement scale (inherent or investigator assigned) of the outcome or dependent variable.

1. DICHOTOMOUS SCALE. One that arranges items into either of two mutually exclusive categories, e.g., Yes/No, Alive/Dead; also termed binary.

2. NOMINAL SCALE. Classification into unordered qualitative categories; e.g. race, religion, and country of birth. Measurements of individual attributes are purely nominal scales, as there is no inherent order to their categories.

3. ORDINAL SCALE. Classification into ordered qualitative categories, e.g. social class (I, II, III, etc.), where the values have a distinct order but their categories are qualitative in that there is no natural (numerical) distance between their possible values.

4. INTERVAL SCALE. An (equal) interval involves assignment of values with a natural distance between them, so that a particular distance (interval) between two values in one region of the scale meaningfully represents the same distance between two values in another region of the scale. Examples include Celsius and Fahrenheit temperature, date of birth.

5. RATIO SCALE. A ratio is an interval scales with a true zero point, so that ratios between values are meaningfully defined. Examples are absolute temperature, weight, height, blood count, distance walked in a given time period, and income, as in each case it is meaningful to speak of one value as being so many times greater or less than another value.[65]

MEASUREMENT THEORY

A theory about how the scores generated by items represent the construct to be measured.[18] See also CLASSICAL TEST THEORY, ITEM RESPONSE THEORY and RASCH MEASUREMENT THEORY and UTILITY THEORY

MEDICATION COMPLIANCE

Typically defined as the extent to which a patient acts in accordance with the prescribed interval and dose of a dosing regimen which is measured over a period of time and reported as a percentage. Although the term adherence is often preferred as it connotes a shared agreement between patients and providers, "compliance" was chosen by ISPOR as the primary term and "adherence" as a synonym based on similar usage by indexing services (e.g. MEDLINE, PubMed).[210]

MENTAL HEALTH

A state of well-being in which every individual realizes his or her own potential, can cope with the normal stresses of life, can work productively and fruitfully, and is able to make a contribution to her or his community; it is manifested by how an individual thinks, feels, and acts when faced with life's situations including handling stress, relating to other people, and making decisions. A mental health problem is a psychiatric disorder that results in a disruption in a person's thinking, feeling, moods, and ability to relate to others. Mental health is not just the absence of mental disorder.[12, 211, 212]

MENTAL ILLNESSES OR MENTAL HEALTH DISORDERS

Diagnosable illnesses that significantly interfere with thought processing abilities, social abilities, emotions and behaviours. Mental illnesses are classified into several broad categories including mood disorders (major depression disorder, bipolar disorder, dysthymia), anxiety disorders (e.g. generalized anxiety disorder, panic disorder, and social phobia), psychotic disorders (e.g. Schizophrenia), cognitive impairment (e.g. Dementia), substance abuse disorders (e.g. alcohol dependency), and disorders of childhood and adolescence (e.g. Attention deficit hyperactivity disorder, childhood anxiety disorder).[213, 214]

META-ANALYSIS

A statistical method to summarize data across studies in order to generate pooled estimates of effects; often the final step when conducting a systematic review when there is a sufficiently high degree of homogeneity of effect across studies to make a pooled estimate meaningful.[215, 216] The most common is an aggregate meta-analysis; other methods are defined below.

1. BAYESIAN HIERARCHICAL META-ANALYSIS: A method that considers prior information to choose different distributions for the between-study standard deviation.[217]

2. INDIVIDUAL PATIENT DATA META-ANALYSIS: Involves obtaining raw data on all patients from each of the studies directly and then re-analyzing them; also termed a pooled analysis.[216]

3. NETWORK META-ANALYSIS: A method in which multiple treatments (that is, three or more) are being compared using both direct comparisons of interventions within randomized controlled trials and indirect comparisons across trials based on a common comparator.[218]

4. META REGRESSION: Tool used in meta-analysis to examine the impact of moderator variables on study effect size using regression-based

techniques.[219]   Here the effects of these variables are estimated using the sample size of the study to weight their contribution and estimate variance.

MINIMAL DETECTABLE CHANGE (MDC)

See CHANGE.

MINIMAL CLINICALLY IMPORTANT DIFFERENCE (MCID)

See CHANGE.

MISSING DATA

A situation that arises commonly in research when study participants fail to complete one or more components of an evaluation, fail to attend an evaluation, or are unavailable for the evaluation because of illness or death. A key feature of missing data is whether the reason for missingness was unrelated to the person such as with equipment failure or inclement weather, or the reason was related to the person. Missing data poses a threat to the validity of research as the people "surviving" to the end of the study with complete data can differ from those starting the study, and the analysis is based on a sample size smaller than planned, reducing statistical power. Different approaches to handling missing data are available but choice is based on the type of missing data. However, the best solution to the missing data problem "is not to have any".[66]

1. IGNORABLE MISSING DATA: Data that are missing at random and the mechanisms that govern the missing data process are unrelated to the parameters to be estimated; there is no need to model the missing data mechanism as part of the estimation process but special techniques will be needed to use these data efficiently.[66]

    a. MISSING COMPLETELY AT RANDOM (MCAR): An assumption made about the nature missing data. Data are assumed to be MCAR when the missing values on the outcome (Y) are unrelated to the value of the outcome (Y) or to the values of any other variables in the data set (Xs). When data are MCAR, the set of people with complete data can be regarded as a simple random subsample from the original set of observations. Studies which measure certain variables for only for a subset of the sample to reduce costs, for example, would have data considered to the MCAR, as would studies with missing data due to equipment, evaluator or administrative error, as examples.[66]

b. MISSING AT RANDOM (MAR): Data are assumed to be missing at random (MAR) when the missing values on the outcome (Y) are unrelated to the value of the outcome (Y) after controlling for the other variables in the analysis. As an example, the MAR assumption would be satisfied if the probability of missing data on a quality of life outcome in a sample of people with cancer depended on a person's severity of gastrointestinal symptoms (none, moderate, severe) but within each category of severity, the probability of missing quality of life is unrelated to quality of life.[66]

2. NON-IGNORABLE MISSING DATA: Data that are not MAR and that the mechanism acting to produce the missing data is non-ignorable. In this instance listwise deletion may be required.[66]

a. NOT MISSING AT RANDOM (NMAR). Data are missing depending on the value of the outcome, such as when patients are too ill or considerably improved and do not attend for evaluation. This type of missing data should be avoided at all costs and ensure that sufficient explanatory information is collected including data from other sources, such as proxies. Being aware of this situation at the design stage will ensure that the protocol is written to permit adequate measurement and follow-up.[66]

MIXED METHODS

Mixed methods research is the type of research in which a researcher or team of researchers combines elements of qualitative and quantitative research approaches (e.g., use of qualitative and quantitative viewpoints, data collection, analysis, inference techniques) for the broad purposes of breadth and depth of understanding and corroboration.[220]

MODEL

Models are the way theories are operationalized in order to develop methods to test hypotheses that arise from theory; they tend to focus on explaining a phenomenon; using the road map analogy (See also THEORY), it is the trip plan that uses the map and a basis for planning.[221, 222] Models can be simple such as the model to derive degrees Farenheight from degree Centigrade ($^{O}F = 32 + 9/5^{O}C$), or complex such as modeling quality of life as an function of personal factors, environmental factors, symptoms, function, and health perception as in the Wilson-Cleary model.[223]

MODERN PSYCHOMETRIC METHODS

Mathematical models that articulate the conditions under which equal interval measurements can be estimated from rating scale data (ordinal response options for a collection of items which are theorized to relate to an underlying construct). Modern psychometrics stress the importance of item response models in which people or patients with a particular level of ability have a probability of responding positively to different questions. There are two general schools of thought, item response theory (IRT) and Rasch measurement, which can be characterized by their approach. As such, when questionnaire data satisfy (fit) the conditions required by these mathematical models, the estimates derived from the models are considered robust. When data do not fit the chosen model, two directions of inquiry are possible. In essence, when the data do not fit the chosen model, the IRT approach is to find a mathematical model that best fits the observed item response data; by contrast, the Rasch measurement approach is to find data that better fit one model (the Rasch model). Thus, it follows that proponents of IRT use a family of item-response models, while proponents of Rasch measurement use only one model (Rasch model). While termed "modern" the mathematical assumptions emerged from work as far back as the 1920s (Thurstone) through to the 1960s (Rasch and Lord).[224, 225]

MORBIDITY

A disease or incidence of disease within a population. Morbidity also refers to adverse effects caused by treatment.[52]

MOTIVATION

The term used to describe the positive construct characterized by openness to experience, energy for daily activities, and having goals and plans for the future. In the context of health, impaired motivation is one the criteria for apathy along with blunting of emotion. A person who lacks motivation, say following a devastating health event, may not necessarily be apathetic if this lack of motivation is a source of distress; if the person is not affected emotionally by lack of motivation, this approaches apathy. Thus, apathy and motivation could be considered to be at opposite ends of an apathy-motivation continuum.[20-23]

MULTIPLE IMPUTATION

A Monte Carlo technique (simulation technique) that replaces each missing datum with a set of m > 1 plausible values. The rn versions of the complete data are analyzed by standard complete-data methods, and the results are combined using simple rules to yield estimates, standard errors, and p-values that formally incorporate missing-data uncertainty.[226]

N

NARRATIVE

Socially constrained forms of action, socially situated performances, and/or ways of acting in and making sense of the world; a form of retrospective meaning-making.[38, 91]

NARRATIVE INQUIRY

A type of qualitative research revolving around an interest in biographical particulars as narrated (orally or written) by the one who lives them.[38, 91]

NARRATIVE REVIEWS

Qualitative summaries of evidence on a specific topic. Because this type of review often does not explicitly describe how the reviewers searched, selected, and appraised the studies included in the review, systematic reviews are increasingly preferred in biomedical journals.[227]

NAY-SAYER

See YEA-SAYER and ACQUIESCENCE BIAS.

NECESSARY

In the context of causal inference, a necessary factor is one that needs to be present for an outcome to be observed; contrasted with sufficient as in "necessary but not sufficient" meaning that the necessary factor cannot act on its own.[42]

NEEDS

What an individual requires to achieve and maintain health and well-being; areas of needs include: physical, emotional, mental health, spiritual, environmental, social, sexual, financial and cultural.[12]

NEEDS ASSESSMENT

A systematic procedure for determining the nature and extent of health needs in a population, the causes and contributing factors to those needs and the human, organizational and community resources which are available to respond to these.[33, 65]

NESTED CASE CONTROL STUDY

Refers to a case-control study that is nested within a cohort study. In this type of study a population is identified and followed over time. At the time the population is identified, baseline data are obtained and this population is followed for a period of years. A case-control study is then conducted using persons in whom a disease develops (cases) and a sample of those in whom the disease did not develop (controls). Note: Only after the disease has developed in some subjects is the case-control study begun.[17]

NETWORK (SOCIAL NETWORK)

Within formal network theory, the term network refers to the ties that connect a specific set of individuals or other social entities such as corporations, groups, or families; the scope and extensiveness of personal networks are used in the measurement of social integration.[69, 228]

NETWORK ANALYSIS

A quantitative way of studying social structure and how the structural properties of the social network affect behaviour; data for social network analysis are derived from the regularities in the patterning of relationships among social entities, which might be people, groups, or organisations.[228]

NEUROTICISM

Individual differences in the tendency to experience chronic negative affect and psychological distress (e.g., tension, depression, frustration, guilt and self-consciousness). Associated cognitive and behavioral styles include irrational thinking, low self-esteem, poor impulse control, somatic complaints and ineffective coping. Neuroticism is the most widely studied trait of the five factor model of personality.[147]

NOMINAL GROUP PROCESS

A structured variant of brain storming using small group discussion to obtain consensus. Each member of the group writes down their ideas on the topic proposed and then, in turn, proposes one for group discussion; the process is repeated until no more ideas are generated and then the ideas are prioritized one by one by the group. The structured process for generating and prioritizing ideas prevents the domination of discussion by a single person, encourages the more passive group members to participate, and results in a set of prioritized solutions or recommendations.[229-231]

NON-INFERIORITY TRIAL

A randomized controlled trial in which the new experimental treatment is compared to a proven active control treatment but the new treatment may not be superior to the active treatment in terms of efficacy, but it may be equivalent. This term has replaced an older term, bioequivalency, or equivalency trial. The objective of a non-inferiority clinical trial is to establish that the effect of the new treatment, when compared to the active control, is not below some pre-stated non-inferiority margin. The null hypothesis is that the control is superior to the experimental treatment group and the alternative hypothesis is the experimental group is not inferior to the control. This non-inferiority margin cannot be greater than the smallest effect size that the active drug would be reliably expected to have compared with placebo in the setting of a placebo-controlled trial.[232]   See also SUPERIORITY TRIAL.

NON-LINEAR

A relationship between two variables that does not follow a straight line; the non-linear relationship may be monotonic (always changing in the same direction) or not (such as a J-shaped curve); to assess the relationship, data from more than 3 time points or categories needs to be available; it can be detected by visual inspection or, in a regression model, it can be tested by fitting a second term for the x variable such as x^2 or x^3 and by verifying whether categories produce results that are similar to those from the regression coefficient (β) from the linear model with only the x variable.[233]

NON-PARAMETRIC METHODS

More correctly termed distribution-free methods, these are statistical techniques that do not depend on specifying the probability distribution from which the sample was drawn. These methods often involve only the ranks of the observations rather than the observations themselves. Examples are Mann-Whitney U test, Wilcoxon's signed rank test and Friedman's two way analysis of variance. These tests are only slightly less powerful than parametric tests which assume a particular population distribution (usually a normal distribution), even when that assumption is true; in the presence of non-normality these tests have greater statistical efficiency (needs less sample size to identify an effect).[3]

NUMBER NEEDED TO HARM

Number of people whose treatment will produce one additional adverse event. It is calculated as the reciprocal of the difference in adverse event rates between two treatment groups. As adverse events can range, Zermansky has suggested separating adverse events and calculating number needed to kill, number needed to disable, number needed to make ill, and number needed to annoy.[65, 234]

NUMBER NEEDED TO TREAT (NNT)

Number of people who need to be treated with the intervention to help one. It is calculated as 1 / difference in risk (of a attaining a positive or preventing a negative outcome) between two treatment groups. Centre for Evidence Based Medicine, Oxford, has a very useful calculator for NNT.[65]

NUMERICAL RATING SCALE (NRS)

NRS Numerical rating scale, commonly from 0 to 10 (11-point scale) or 1 to 10 (10-point scale); usually, only the two extreme categories are labeled, for example, ''No pain at all'' and ''Worst imaginable pain.'' NRS may need to be explained or shown on paper to the patient, who responds by indicating a number, in which case this is referred to as a Visual NRS (VNRS) or VNS.[235]

O

OBSERVER REPORTED OUTCOME (ObsRO)

An outcome that is assessed by a person, not necessarily with any expert training, who reports on observed behavior of person who cannot respond for themselves; observers cannot report on how another person's feels (pain, fatigue) but only on what they are observed to do (cry, self-care, walk etc.).[55]

OCCUPATIONAL THERAPY

The art and science of enabling engagement in everyday living, through occupation; of enabling people to perform the occupations that foster health and well-being; and of enabling a just and inclusive society so that all people may participate to their potential in the daily occupations of life.[236]

ODDS

Ratio of the probability of having an event to the probability of not having the event; odds of 2:1 indicates that 2/3 persons will have an event and 1/3 will not.[65]

ODDS RATIO

Ratio of two odds: the odds associated with people with the factor under study relative to the odds for people without the factor under study.[65]

ONTOLOGY

Model of what is known in a domain.[5]

OPENNESS TO EXPERIENCE

One of the "big five" personality traits, reflecting individual differences in the "breadth, depth and permeability of consciousness, and in the recurrent need to enlarge and examine experience". Highly open people are frequently viewed as imaginative, sensitive to art and beauty, emotionally differentiated, behaviorally flexible, intellectually curious and liberal in values; openness is inversely related to authoritarianism/dogmatism and need for closure. Openness shows a maturational trend, increasing from early adolescence through the 20s, then gradually declining.[237, 238]

OPPORTUNITY COSTS

The benefits lost because the next-best alternative was not selected.[180]

ORDINAL

A type of discrete data where the values fall into a limited number of categories each with an inherent order; ordinal outcome data can be efficiently modeled using ordinal regression through the proportional odds model or cumulative odds model.[239, 240]

OUTCOME

In the context of health, an aspect of an individual's physical, emotional, mental or social health that is expected to change owing to a deliberate intervention or to vary in the presence of another personal, health or environmental factor. Kerr White coined the term the 5D's for health outcomes (death, disease, discomfort, disability, dissatisfaction).[241] A more modern list would be mortality (death), morbidity (disease), disability (which encompasses discomfort using ICF framework), dissatisfaction (with the process or the outcome), and cost (or the 6D, destitution which could be of the person or the health care system).[242]

P

P-VALUE

The probability of obtaining a given result by chance alone.[4]

PALLIATIVE CARE

The active total care offered to a person and that person's family when it is recognized that the illness is no longer curable, in order to concentrate on the person's quality of life and the alleviation of distressing symptoms. The focus of palliative care is neither to hasten nor postpone death. It provides relief from pain and other distressing symptoms and integrates the psychological and spiritual aspects of care. It offers a support system to help relatives and friends cope during an individual's illness and with their bereavement.[187]

PANEL STUDY

A combination of cross-sectional and cohort methods in which the investigator conducts a series of cross-sectional studies of the same individuals or study sample. This method of study permits changes in one variable to be related to changes in other variables.[7]

PAPER ADAPTIVE TEST

Version of a computerized adaptive test where the response choices are presented in a printed format; in many clinical situations, this format is more feasible. An example of this format can be found in a paper by Higgins, for a ClinRO for upper extremity function post-stroke.[243]

PARTICIPATION

In the context of health, it is involvement in a life situation; a component of the umbrella term for function as defined by the WHO's ICF which comprises body function and structure, activity and participation; participation reflects the societal perspective on functioning and covers domains of interpersonal relationships, major life areas (education, work, and economic life), and community, social and civic life.[7]

PARTICIPATION RESTRICTION

In the context of health, a problems an individual may experience in involvement in a life situation; problems can be in capacity or in performance; it is a component of the umbrella term for disability as defined by the WHO's ICF which comprises additionally, impairments and activity limitations.[7]

PARTICIPATORY RESEARCH

A methodology that is based on the co-creation of new knowledge by researchers working in equitable partnerships with those who are most impacted by the issue under study, or those who must act on the research results; this method aims to achieve a balance between the needs of scientists to develop valid and generalizable knowledge and the need to provide benefits to the community being researched.[244]

PATH ANALYSIS

A method of analysis involving assumptions about the direction of causal relationships between linked sequences and configurations of variables. This permits the analyst to construct and test the appropriateness of alternative models (in the form of a path diagram) of the causal relations that may exist within the array of variables included in the finite system studied. Identification of the less probable sequences of causal pathways may permit them to be eliminated from further consideration.[65]

PATIENT-CENTERED CARE

Health care that is compassionate, empathetic, and focussed on the patient's own worldview, goals, preferences, values, and needs.[245-247]

PATIENT-CENTERED OUTCOMES

Outcomes that patients care about: survival, symptoms, function, and health-related quality of life.[248]

PATIENT-CENTERED OUTCOMES RESEARCH

Research that helps people and their caregivers communicate and make informed health care decisions, allowing their voices to be heard in assessing the value of health care options. This research answers patient-centered questions such as: (i) what a person can expect from treatment; (ii) what options are available and potential benefits and harms; (iii) what can be done to improve the outcomes that are most important; (iv) how to make the best decisions about health and healthcare.[246]

PATIENT ENGAGEMENT

A strategy to engage people who represent the population of interest and other relevant stakeholders, into the research process, including: designing the study, selecting measures, enhancing subject recruitment, interpreting findings, and/or disseminating study findings; through the active incorporation of perspectives beyond those of the researchers, the research and its results have more assurance that they will be patient-centered, relevant to the intended users of the research findings, and that the findings can be effectively disseminated.[249]

PATIENT REPORTED EXPERIENCE MEASURES (PREMs)

Measures related to patient-centered care that cover aspects of the structure and processes of care as experienced by the patient and not interpreted by any other person. Dimensions of the patient experience covered by PREMs include respect for patients' values and preferences; provision of information, communication and education; coordination of care; involvement of family; emotional support; physical comfort; preparation for discharge, continuity and transitions in care; and access. In the hospital context, PREMs cover aspects of care such as communication and responsiveness of health professionals, cleanliness and quietness of the environment, pain management, and adequacy of discharge information. PREMs are distinct from measures of satisfaction as the latter is strongly affected by expectations and outcomes.[250-254]

PATIENT-REPORTED OUTCOMES (PROs)

A measurement of any aspect of a patient's health that comes directly from the patient without interpretation of the patient's responses by a physician or anyone else[2, 55]. A distinction can be made between those outcomes for which no other interpretation is valid, such as the rating of symptoms or difficulty in carrying out an activity, and those outcomes where verification is possible. For example, the patient can be a good source of information on limitations in physical function, but if need be, the information reported on could be verified by observed performance. The term Self-reported Outcome (SRO) would better represent this type of construct.[255]

PEARSON PRODUCT MOMENT CORRELATION

See CORRELATION COEFFICIENT.

PERFORMANCE

Execution of a task or activity in the current environment in contrast to capacity which is in a standard environment such as a clinic or laboratory; terms used by the WHO to define function and disability in the context of the ICF framework.[7] Despite this definition from the disability perspective, performance or performance-based is often used for outcomes that are assessed by having the person "perform" a test, such as the Six minute walk test (6MWT); these types of tests are termed Performance Rated Outcomes (PerfRO or PerfO).[55, 255] Within the disability framework, this type of test would be considered a test of capacity and whether the person walks outside in their community or around their house would be considered performance.

PERFORMANCE RATED OUTCOME (PerfRO or PerfO)

See PERFORMANCE

PERSONALIZED MEDICINE

An emerging practice of medicine that uses an individual's genetic profile to guide decisions made in regard to the prevention, diagnosis, and treatment of disease. Knowledge of a person's genetic profile can help identify the type and dose of medication or therapy best suited to the individual or to a certain group of people. Personalized medicine is being advanced through data from the Human Genome Project.[30]

PERSON CENTERED APPROACH

Ways of commissioning, providing and organising services rooted in listening to what people want, to help them live in their communities as they choose. These approaches work to use resources flexibly, designed around what is important to an individual from their own perspective and work to remove any cultural and organisational barriers. People are not simply placed in pre-existing services and expected to adjust, rather the service strives to adjust to the person.[12]

PHASE I CLINICAL STUDY

The first of three sets of studies in the sequence of testing of new drugs by the U.S. Food and Drug Administration prior to their approval for use in the general or specific populations. Phase I trials are small pharmacological studies of 20-80 patients that examine toxic and pharmacological effects.[17]

PHASE II CLINICAL STUDY

The second of three sets of studies in the sequence of testing of new drugs by the U.S. Food and Drug Administration prior to their approval for use in the general or specific populations. Phase II studies are clinical investigations of 100-200 patients to specifically examine the safety and efficacy of new drugs.[17]

PHASE III CLINICAL STUDY

The third of three sets of studies in the sequence of testing of new drugs by the U.S. Food and Drug Administration prior to their approval for use in the general or specific populations. Phase III studies are large scale, often multi-centered randomized controlled trials to examine the effectiveness and related safety of new drugs.[17]

PHASE IV CLINICAL STUDY

Postmarketing surveillance used to monitor new drugs that is conducted after the drug has been approved for use by the public. The goal of Phase IV monitoring is to identify adverse effects such as carcinogenesis and teratogenesis that are so small or infrequent that they may not be evident for many years, even in very large Phase III trials.[17]

PHENOMENOLOGY

A complex, multifaceted philosophy proposing that legitimate knowledge comes from a careful description of ordinary conscious experience of everyday life (termed the life-world) by a description of 'things' as one experiences them through perception (hearing, seeing, etc.), believing, remembering, deciding, feeling, judging, evaluating etc.; this philosophy challenges the scientific realism approach that genuine legitimate knowledge can come only from 'things' or from 'what is' and focuses on the knowledge through the meaning of 'things'.[38]

PHYSICAL ACTIVITY

In the context of exercise, physical activity is defined as body movements produced by skeletal muscle action resulting in increased energy expenditure.[127, 128] These movements occur as part of everyday life. See also EXERCISE.

PHYSICAL ENVIRONMENT

Consists of the natural environment (i.e., plants, atmosphere, weather, and topography) and the built environment (i.e., buildings, spaces, transportation systems, and products that are created or modified by people). Physical environments can consist of particular individual or institutional settings, such as homes, worksites, schools, health care settings, or recreational settings. Surrounding neighbourhoods and related community areas where individuals live, work, travel, play, and conduct their other daily activities are elements of the physical environment.[256]

PILOT STUDY

A small scale test of the methods and procedures to be used on a larger scale if the pilot study demonstrates that these methods and procedures can work. In this context "capacity to work" relates to processes as well as to deriving an estimate of the extent to which the intervention group changes (potential for efficacy) as, if no change is observed, perhaps pursuing this avenue of intervention is not warranted. A pilot study does not test a hypothesis, however, it is always beneficial to have a control group (even if there is no intent to do a between group comparison) as "nothing improves the appearance of an intervention so much as the absence of a control group". Pilot studies tend to overestimate intervention effects owing to a phenomenon Cronbach called super realization bias referring to the observation that it is easier to achieve optimal processes and outcomes with smaller studies as each participant gets more attention that can be afforded in larger studies.[3, 5, 257-262]

PLACEBO

Any therapy (or that component of any therapy) that is intentionally or knowingly used for its nonspecific, psychological, or psycho-physiological, therapeutic effect or that is used for a presumed specific therapeutic effect on a patient, symptom, or illness but is without specific activity for the conditions being treated.[263]

PLACEBO-CONTROLLED

When a substance or procedure without any specific activity for the condition being treated is used as a control in an experimental study.[263]

PLACEBO EFFECT

The nonspecific psychological or psycho-physiological therapeutic effect produced by a placebo.[263]

PLATFORM TRIAL

An extension of the adaptive trial design which has a broad aim to identify the best treatment for a health conditions by simultaneously investigating multiple treatments. The design requires specialized statistical methods for allocating patients and analyzing results. The focus is on the health condition rather than any particular experimental therapy. Platform trials use decision rules (e.g. based on the likelihood of a treatment benefit or of success in a future confirmatory trial to determine when a given treatment regimen has demonstrated sufficient efficacy to "graduate" from the trial and to the next stage in development or to implementation. Bayesian probabilities can also be used to determine when a treatment should be eliminated from the trial, or from subgroups of patients, because it is no longer sufficiently participating. Its advantage is that several interventions can be tested but less effective ones can be eliminated so people can then be assigned to more promising interventions. While conceived for the evaluation of pharmaceuticals, different types of interventions could be tested using this design.[264]

POLYCHORIC CORRELATION

See CORRELATION COEFFICIENT.

POLYTOMOUS

A categorical variable with 3 or more categories.[5]

POOLED ANALYSIS

See META-ANALYSIS: INDIVIDUAL PATIENT DATA META-ANALYSIS.

POSITIVE PREDICTIVE VALUE (PPV)

The percentage of persons deemed positive on a test who actually have the condition of interest. To be distinguished from sensitivity which is the proportion of people with the condition of interest who tested positive. The PPV provides results that are most directly relevant for the decision to use or not a given measure.[265]

POST-HOC COMPARISON

Analyses of contrasts not explicitly planned at the start of a study but suggested after an examination of the data. Optimally, this is done only when a global effect is detected in the data otherwise the results are less believable.[3]

POST-TEST

In the context of a randomized trial, a post-test can be done to estimate effectiveness of an intervention as, because of randomization, the groups have the same baseline distribution. Alternately, in the context of quality of life research, quality of life outcomes cannot be assessed when people are acutely ill but the long-term impact of an intervention targeting quality of life is relevant; here only the post-test value is analysed as the pre-test value was not obtained.[266, 267]

POSTERIOR PROBABILITY

The probability of an event or observation calculated based on the existing data. In clinical decision making, it is the probability of disease given a symptom. In group based trajectory analysis, it is the probability a person belongs to a particular longitudinal pattern of behaviour defined from the data.[65]

POWER

Power is the strength a study has to detect a difference between two treatments or two levels of a factor, if these do in fact differ; it is expressed as 1—probability of making type II error (1-β), risk an investigator is willing to take to say two treatments do not differ when they do. Underpowered studies may falsely conclude that an intervention is not effective, when in fact it may well be; thus, it is important when looking at small clinical studies to examine the estimate of effect and its confidence interval, rather than the p-value alone.[17]

PRECISION

Precision is an index of how closely results can be duplicated from one measurement to the next. As such, it may be a useful summary statistic when applied to assays, but it does not (1) differentiate between inter- and intra-rater reliability, or (2) incorporate the concept of reliability reflecting the ability of the tool to differentiate among people. In the context of statistics, it is a term applied to the likely spread of estimates of a parameter in a statistical model; measured by the standard error of the estimator; this can be decreased, and hence precision increased, by using a larger sample size.[3, 4]

PREDICTIVE VALIDITY

The extent to which the value on a test or measure under study predicts future performance or events. Ideally, predictive validity is tested on a dataset that is different than the one used to develop the test or measure.[2]

PREFERENCE

Preference is the desirability for a particular health outcome or health state.[268]

PREFERENCE-BASED MEASURES

Preference-based measures are a subset of HRQL measures which can be generic or disease-specific. Derived from economic, decision-analytic, and psychometric traditions, these measures have a central concept that individuals have quantifiable preferences for health outcomes. Different methods are used to elicit preferences but all result in a single number for HRQL anchored in death at 0 and perfect health at 1.0. These scores permit the combining of mortality and morbidity and the calculation of quality-adjusted life years (QALY), which can be used to make comparisons across health states, illnesses and populations. Recently, disease specific preference based measures have been developed raising concerns as to how preferences are obtained and who provides preferences, the general population or people with specific health conditions.[269-271]

PREFERENCES FOR CARE

The wishes, views and choices of individuals about their language and communication, beliefs, personal care, where they wish to live, how their independence and potential can be maximised and how they should be treated.[12]

PREFERENCE WEIGHT

A numerical judgement describing preferences or utility as function of specific variables.[180]

PREVALENCE

The number of affected persons present in the population at a specific time. When compared to the number of persons in the population at that time, the correct term is prevalence rate.[17]

PREVALENCE STUDY

See CROSS SECTIONAL STUDY.

PREVALENT CASES

At the start of a study, it is the number of people who already have the condition under study; continued follow-up of the sample will yield additional cases, termed incident cases; it is important to distinguish prevalent cases from incident cases in studies which may contain both.[52]

PREVENTION

Actions that prevent disease occurrence or are aimed at five levels of preventions (as defined below)[5, 105] recognizing that effective prevention strategies interact and operate across levels. Eliminating or minimizing the impact of disease and disability or retarding the process of disease and disability.

1. PRIMORDIAL PREVENTION consists of establishing conditions or actions to minimize health hazards to prevent the emergence of risk factors that may then be the subject of primary prevention, in other words preventing the risk factor itself. Usually accomplished through health policy; smoking bans in public places and establishment of green space in a community are examples.

2. PRIMARY PREVENTION aims at preventing the initial occurrence of a disorder by personal and community efforts, such as increasing physical activity and improving nutritional status, decreasing environmental risks, improving water quality and immunizing against communicable diseases. It is considered the core task of public health and includes health promotion.

3. SECONDARY PREVENTION aims at reducing the prevalence of disease by shortening its duration. For diseases that have no cure, secondary prevention strategies will aim to increase survival and quality of life. However this will also increase the prevalence of the disease. Screening programs are examples of secondary prevention strategies, as are most clinical interventions.

4. TERTIARY PREVENTION aims to prevent the sequelae of health conditions including relapses, emergence of new chronic conditions and disability. Provision of effective

rehabilitation is considered one of the main methods of tertiary prevention.

5. QUATERNARY PREVENTION consists of actions to identify patients at risk of over diagnosis or overtreatment and to protect people from excessive medical intervention thereby preventing iatrogenesis. Identifying people at risk for polypharmacy and establishing medical review program is an example of quaternary prevention.[272, 273]

PRIMARY CANCER

Original cancer; to be distinguished from secondary cancers which may arise as a consequence of treatment for primary cancers.[52]

PRIMARY CARE PROVIDER

Health professional who manages a person's health care over time. A primary care provider is able to give a wide range of care, including prevention and treatment, discuss treatment choices, and can refer a patient to a specialist.[52]

PRIMARY HEALTH CARE

Essential health care based on practical, scientifically sound and socially acceptable methods and technology that is made universally accessible to individuals and families in the community through their full participation and at a cost that the community and country can afford to maintain at every stage of their development in the spirit of self-reliance and self-determination.[274]

PRIMARY PREVENTION

See PREVENTION.

PROBABILITY

The likelihood of an event; in the context of a health event, it is usually expressed as the proportion of those experiencing the event among those who are at risk for experiencing the event.[275]

PROFILE

In the context of health measurement, a profile is a collection of items which are summarized to yield separate values for the different domains. The well-known and widely used SF-36 is an example of a health profile as 8 scores are generated for general health, physical function, pain, vitality, mental health, social function, physical role and emotional role. Health profiles do not indicate the relative importance attached to the various dimensions covered.[18]

PROPENSITY SCORES

Conditional probability of exposure to a treatment given specific observed covariates[5, 276, 277]; propensity scoring is an efficient way of managing multiple variables that impact on exposure variables without having to adjust for each variable separately. A propensity score can be estimated for each individual by fitting a logistic regression model where the exposure takes the place of the outcome variable, and the measured confounding variables are included as explanatory variables. The predicted exposure probabilities from this model are the estimated propensity scores, which by definition all lie between zero and one. Other models can be used by logistic regression is the most common.[278] Consider the situation where an investigator wishes to know whether people with chronic respiratory disease who exercise have better HRQL than people who do not exercise, however, many variables are associated both with the exposure (exercise) and the outcome (HRQL), too many to realistically use in a statistical model. Propensity scoring can be used to estimate an individual's propensity to exercise and this score can be used for matching, adjustment, or stratification.

PROPORTIONAL MORTALITY

The proportion of deaths caused by a specific disease: (# of deaths / total deaths) X 100.[17] Interpretation of this parameter is not straightforward as change or differences can result from an increase or excess in one cause of death or a deficiency in another. In many countries, the proportional mortality associated with chronic diseases has increased dramatically as deaths due to infectious diseases have fallen.[279]

PROSPECTIVE

Examining events over a period of time beginning in the present and continuing into the future. This type of observation is applied in certain types of cohort studies.[17]

PSYCHOMETRICS

Refers to a field of study and practice that deals with the theories and techniques of psychological measurement. The major psychometric tasks include development of assessment models, development of psychological instruments, designing and conducting assessments, and then analysis and interpretation of measurements. Modern psychometrics incorporates the measurement theories of Classical Test Theory (CTT), Item Response Theory (IRT), Rasch Measurement Theory (RMT), and Utility Theory.[280] See also CLASSICAL TEST THEORY, ITEM RESPONSE THEORY (IRT), RASCH MEASUREMENT THEORY (RMT), AND UTILITY THEORY.

PUBLIC HEALTH

A social and political concept aimed at improving health, prolonging life and improving the quality of life among whole populations through health promotion, disease prevention and other forms of health intervention. Public health is based on a comprehensive understanding of the ways in which lifestyles and living conditions determine health status, and a recognition of the need to mobilize resources and make sound investments in policies, programs and services which create, maintain and protect health.[105]

PURPOSIVE SAMPLING

A method of sampling to choose sites, cases, or other objects of inquiry for research because they are thought to provide information critical to understanding some process or concept or for testing or elaborating some established theory; the object of inquiry may be chosen based on prior knowledge that it is extreme, typical, deviant, or otherwise unique, or particularly revealing; nevertheless some relevant criteria are established and then the object is chosen because it meets criteria; also called criterion-based selection.[38]

Q

QUALITATIVE EVALUATION

A variety of approaches to evaluating or determining the merit or worth of programs, policies, projects, or technologies making use of qualitative methods for generating data such as unstructured interviewing, observation, document analysis and non-statistical means of analysing and presenting the data.[38]

QUALITATIVE RESEARCH

A situated activity that locates the observer in the world using a set of interpretive and material practices that make the world visible; qualitative researcher emphasizes the qualities of entities and on processes and meanings that are not experimentally examined or measured (if measured at all) in terms of quantity, amount, intensity, or frequency. In contrast to quantitative research that emphasizes the measurement and analysis of causal relationships between variables, qualitative research emphasizes the processes linking the variables together. Qualitative researchers stress the socially constructed nature of reality, the intimate relationship between the researcher and what is studied, and the situational constraints that shape inquiry. They seek answers to questions that stress how social experience is created and given meaning. Qualitative methods make use of a series of current and historical representations such field notes, interviews, conversations, photographs, artefacts, cultural texts and productions, recordings, and memos to the self; diverse methods are also employed to see the world such as case study, introspection, life story interview, observation, interaction, and personal experience that describe routine and problematic moments and meanings in individuals' lives.[38, 91]

QUALITY ADJUSTED LIFE YEARS (QALYs)

A measure of health outcome which assigns to each period of time a weight, ranging from 0 to 1, corresponding to the health related quality of life during that period, where a weight of 1 corresponds to optimal health and a weight of 0 corresponds to a health state judged equivalent to death; these are then aggregated across time periods.[180]

QUALITY MEASURE

Quantitative indicators that reflect the degree to which care is consistent with the best available, evidence-based, clinical standards.[52]

QUALITY OF CARE

The degree to which health services for individuals and populations increase the likelihood of desired health outcomes and are consistent with current professional knowledge.[52]

QUALITY OF CARE AT END OF LIFE

Satisfaction the care received at end of life; a factor that may influence quality of dying and death and quality of life at the end of life, but is conceptually and operationally unique.[281]

QUALITY OF DEATH

A death that is free from avoidable distress and suffering for patients, families, and their caregivers; in general accord with the patients' and families' wishes; and reasonably consistent with clinical, cultural, and ethical standards.[282]

QUALITY OF DYING

Personal evaluation of the dying experience as a whole, including a subjective evaluation of concepts according to expectations and values.[283]

QUALITY OF DYING AND DEATH

The degree to which a person's preferences for dying and the moment of death agree with observations of how the person actually died as reported by others.[281]

QUALITY OF LIFE (QOL)

A term often used erroneously to refer to health-related quality of life or health status, but is broader than just health and includes components of material comforts, health and personal safety, relationships, learning, creative expression, opportunity to help and encourage others, participation in public affairs, socializing, and leisure. The WHO has defined quality of life as individuals' perception of their position in life in the context of the culture in which they live and in relation to their goals, expectations, standards and concerns. In the context of health research, quality of life goes beyond a description of health status, but rather is a reflection of the way that people perceive and react to their health status and to other, nonmedical aspects of their lives. According to Aristotle, quality of life would be the best kind of life, the happiest life, which is the life of virtue comprising: (i) intellectual or theoretical contemplation including scientific activity, considered the primary form of happiness; and (ii) practical or moral virtue including courage, moderation, generosity, and justice, the secondary from of virtue. In a modern context this would imply that quality of life is a life where one needs to think or contemplate aspects of life engagement and then act in a moral way or, in other words, be both smart and nice.[110, 284-287]

QUALITY OF LIFE IN ANIMALS (QOL- ANIMAL)

A state of an animal's life as perceived by [it] at any one point in time. It is experienced as a sense of well-being which involves the balance between negative and positive affective states and any cognitive evaluation of these, where the animal has the capacity. To some extent, QOL can be predicted by the fulfilment of basic and species specific health, social and environmental needs (and individual preferences for these) and is reflected in the animal's health and behaviour. Animal welfare is a concept closely related to animal QOL and has been assessed in farm animals using the five freedoms: (i) freedom from hunger and thirst; (ii) freedom from pain, injury, and disease; (iii) freedom from discomfort; (iv) freedom from fear and distress; and (v) freedom to express normal behavior.[288] In pets, QOL has focused mainly on behavioral and physical health parameters, although these freedoms would also apply.[178, 289, 290] See also HEALTH RELATED QUALITY OF LIFE OF ANIMALS

QUALITY OF LIFE AT THE END OF LIFE

The experience of living a satisfactory life in the face of terminal illness; focuses on functional status or the fulfillment of needs essential to living even when a person is near death, an emphasis that may or may not be recognized by patients, loved ones, or caregivers.[281]

QUESTIONNAIRE

A term often used to describe a patient-reported outcome or other collection of self-reported items. In the context of modern measurement theory, a questionnaire would be better used to describe a method of gathering data from study subjects on personal and environmental characteristics.

R

RANDOMIZATION

A process of allocation of individuals to groups by chance. It ensures that the probability of being assigned to any group is known in advance of the study and is the same for every person. As a result, differences between the intervention and control groups are random. In large sample sizes groups are similar at the start if the study on both known and unknown variables. No other methodological procedure can accomplish this. Statistically it accounts for uncertainty for unmeasured differences and it also ensures that personal judgement and investigator preferences do not influence allocation. Randomization follows a pre-determined plan usually devised as an aid of a computer program.[5, 56]

RANDOMIZED CLINICAL (CONTROLLED) TRIAL

An experimental study design in which members of a target population are assigned by a random process to two or more study groups. These groups are then followed over time in parallel and are compared on the pre-specified end-point at study end. RCTs aim to evaluate deliberate interventions, often innovations in treatment. This design provides strongest evidence for the benefits or risks of a treatment; the comparison group can be either placebo, the current standard treatment (which may be none), or an active alternative (such as exercise vs. drug therapy), termed a pragmatic trial.[242]

RARE DISEASE ASSUMPTION

An assumption that the disease or outcome understudy is rare in the population studied. This assumption must be met in order for approximations to validly estimate the desired parameter. For example, only when the disease is rare does prevalence approximate the incidence rate multiplied by the average duration of disease ($P = I * D$). The odds ratio (OR) is approximately equal to the incidence rate ratio (IRR) or relative risk (RR) under the rare disease assumption, unless incidence density sampling is used as in a case control study. In epidemiological studies, outcomes are considered rare if they occur in under 2% of the population. Logistic regression is used to analyse data that are binary and this analysis yields the OR, although the RR is usually the parameter of interest. When the outcome is not rare, the OR will over estimate the RR. There is nothing wrong using with reporting the OR but it must be interpreted as an OR and not as an RR.[65]

RASCH ANALYSIS

A method of analyzing data according to the Rasch model, to identify whether or not adding the scores from a collection of items is justified in the data. This is called the test of fit between the data and the model. If the invariance of responses across different groups of people does not hold, then taking the total score to characterize a person is not justified. Of course, data never fit the model perfectly, and it is important to consider the fit of data to the model with respect to the uses to be made of the total scores. If the data do fit the model adequately for the purpose, then the Rasch analysis also linearises the total score, which is bounded by 0 and the maximum score on the items, into measurements. The linearised value is the location of the person on the unidimensional continuum—the value is called a parameter in the model and there can be only one number in a unidimensional framework. This parameter can then be used in analysis of variance and regression more readily than the raw total score, which has floor and ceiling effects.[224, 225]

RASCH MEASUREMENT THEORY

An experimental measurement paradigm based on strong measurement theory providing an evidence base for the extent to which a set of the items form a real measure. The ordering of the categories of the rating scales is tested empirically, and if ordering is not met, further experimentation is required before inferences from the ratings are made.[224, 225]

RASCH MODEL

The Rasch model, named for the Danish mathematician Georg Rasch (1901-1980), is a probabilistic model used to specify an observed rating of a person on a variable of interest as a function of the ability of the person and the difficulty of the items used to derive the rating, where both are defined by their location on continuum from least (easiest) to most (hardest). This model is widely used in health outcome measurement as a way of transforming dichotomous or ordinal response categories onto a linear scale with interval-like properties. It is based on a logit transformation of the probability of response to a particular item; an item that 50% of respondents pass or endorse has a logit of 0. A scale that defines the full spectrum of a construct will range from -4 to +4 logits, corresponding to ± 4 standard deviations defining the full range of a standard normal distribution. People at the low end of the logit scale have less ability whereas people at the high end have more ability; correspondingly, items at the low end are easy to pass or endorse, items at the high end are difficulty to pass or endorse.

Items that fit a Rasch model would form a measure with a total score that is sufficient to determine that person's ability on the underlying construct. When the data derived from observed ratings do not fit the underlying linear and hierarchical model, an investigation as to the source of error needs to be initiated. An item may be poorly worded: "Are you unconcerned with many things?"; or not understood: "Would you consider yourself apathetic?". The categories of response may need to be redefined so that the respondents are better able to distinguish between them. The solution to the problem of poor item fit needs to be resolved with substantive, empirical and experimental input. The analysis cannot reveal the source of the problem, only the location of the problem. That the data fit the Rasch model is only a necessary condition, it is not sufficient to define the construct, this assumption requires theoretical support. Post hoc adjustments of responses to fit the Rasch model are excellent exploratory tools and may be necessary in some cases before making other relevant interpretations, but they need to be backed up by relevant experimental evidence.[224, 225]

RATE

A measure of the frequency of the occurrence of an outcome or event in a defined population and in a specified period of time. The rate is usually expressed as a number per unit population to facilitate interpretation. In epidemiology, the denominator for rates is person time. All rates are ratios; some rates are proportions where the numerator is contained within the denominator. A rate with person time as the denominator would not be a proportion.[5, 291]

RATING SCALE

A scale where values for health states are measured when people assign a number to various conditions on a numerical scale (e.g.0.0-1.0 or 0-100). The highest number on the scale corresponds to the best health imaginable and the lowest number is the worst health imaginable. Health states are ranked on the scale relative to each other and the intervals between the states match the strength of preference between the states.[181] See also VISUAL ANALOG SCALE and NUMERIC RATING SCALE and VERBAL RATING SCALE

RATIO

A ratio is a value obtained by dividing one quantity by another. Both numerator and denominator can be in different units.[5]

RECALL BIAS

A deviation from the truth arising from differential recall of past events for groups of people being compared; in a case-control, the recall of events is often enhanced in cases compared to controls and this may lead to overestimating a relationship between an effect and an outcome.[17]

RECEIVER OPERATING CHARACTERISTICS CURVE (ROC)

A ROC curve is a graph that plots true positive rates against false positive rates for a series of cut-off values on a test, or in other words, graphically displays the trade-off between sensitivity and specificity for each cut-off value. An ideal cut-off might give the test the highest possible sensitivity with the lowest possible false positive rate (i.e., highest specificity). This is the point lying geometrically closest to the top-left corner of the graph (where the ideal cut-off value with 100% sensitivity and specificity would be plotted). Picking the ideal cut-off score is, to some extent, dependent on the clinical context, that is the purpose for which the test will be used. The area under an ROC curve can be used as an overall estimate of its discriminating ability and sometimes is expressed as accuracy. The area under the ROC curve is equal to the probability that a test correctly classifies patients as true positives or true negatives. Greater areas under the curve indicate higher accuracy. To further clarify, a discriminant test might have an area under the curve of 0.7 while a nondiscriminant test has an area under the curve of 0.5.[292]

RECOVERY

The process of getting back to or regaining health or a normal condition after an illness, injury or a period of difficulty.[92]

RECOVERY (MENTAL HEALTH)

The personal process that people with mental health conditions experience in gaining control, meaning and purposes in their lives with the ultimate aim of living a satisfying, hopeful, and contributing life, even when mental health problems and mental illnesses cause ongoing limitations. Recovery involves different things for different people. For some, recovery means the complete absence of the symptoms of mental illness. For others, recovery means living a full life in the community while learning to live with ongoing symptoms.[293-295]

RECOVERY (POST-OPERATIVE)

An energy-requiring process of returning to normality and wholeness as defined by comparative standards, achieved by regaining control over physical, psychological, social, and habitual functions, which results in returning to preoperative levels of independence/dependence in activities of daily living and an optimum level of psychological well-being.[296]

REFLECTIVE CONSTRUCT

See CONCEPTUAL MODEL.

REGRESSION COEFFICIENT (β)

A parameter indicating the change or difference in the outcome (dependent or y variable) corresponding to a one unit change or difference in the explanatory (independent or x) variable. In a linear relationship, this is the slope of the line that relates values of x to values of y; testing whether the slope differs from 0 can be done by dividing the slope parameter (β) by its standard error which is the equivalent to a t-test.[3, 233] See also BETA COEFFICIENT.

REHABILITATION

The health strategy that applies and integrates approaches to optimize a person's capacity, through strengthening the resources of the person, to enable and maintain optimal functioning, and ultimately to enhance the health aspects quality of life. Rehabilitation is applied over the course of a health condition, to all age groups, along and across the continuum of care from hospitals, rehabilitation facilities and in the community, and across sectors including health, education, labor and social affairs with the goal to enable persons with health conditions experiencing or likely to experience disability to achieve and maintain optimal functioning. In this context rehabilitation is based on the WHO's integrative model of functioning, disability, and health (ICF).[297]

1. PULMONARY REHABILITATION: Is an evidence-based, multidisciplinary and comprehensive intervention for patients with chronic respiratory diseases who are symptomatic and often have decreased daily life activities. Integrated into the individualized treatment of the patient, pulmonary rehabilitation is designed to reduce symptoms, optimize functional status, increase participation, and reduce health care costs through stabilizing or reversing systemic manifestations of the disease.[298]

2. CANCER REHABILITATION: Cancer rehabilitation involves helping a person with cancer achieve maximum physical, social, psychological, and vocational functioning within the limits imposed by the disease and its treatment along the continuum of their cancer care.[299]

RELATIVE EFFECTIVENESS

The ratio of two estimates of effectiveness such as ratio of two effect sizes.[50, 300]

RELATIVE RISK

Typically, the ratio of the risk of disease in exposed individuals to the risk of disease in non-exposed individuals. Relative risk can also be defined as the probability of an event or health outcome occurring in exposed individuals compared to the probability of an event or health outcome occurring in non-exposed individuals.[17] It is usually the parameter of interest in longitudinal or cohort studies and is approximated by the odds ratio from a logistic regression model only when the outcome is rare.

RELIABILITY

The extent to which scores for objects of measurement (people or biophysical entities) that have not changed are the same for repeated measurement under several conditions: for example, using different sets of items from the same PROs (internal consistency), over time (test-retest), by different persons on the same occasion (inter-rater) or by the same persons (i.e., raters or responders) on different occasions (intra-rater). It is expressed as the proportion of the total variance in the measurements arising from a "true" differences among objects of measurement where total variance consists of true variation (the variation of interest) and error variation (which includes random error as well as systematic error). Reliability is often used synonymously with reproducibility, stability, consistency or agreement, recognizing that these terms may not be as precisely defined.[4, 46, 199]

RESERVE

Physiological and functional resources an individual has to call upon to meet health challenges[301] ; it can be measured by the difference between capacity (what the person can maximally do) and performance (what they do in everyday activities) and represents the latent or dormant abilities that can be called upon in times of perceived need. At the level of the brain, distinction is made between brain and cognitive reserve with brain reserve considered as the potential ability of the brain to cope with neuronal damage and is measured through the structural aspects such as brain size and synapse count; cognitive reserve is the ability to optimise and maximize performance through recruitment of brain networks and/or compensation by alternative cognitive strategies. Cognitive reserve is thought to be built through intensive cognitive stimulation, particularly in childhood, and is related to education, occupation, intelligence and leisure activities.[301-303]

RESILIENCE

The intrinsic ability of a system to adjust its functioning prior to, during, or following changes and disturbances. Resilient systems have been defined as those that (1) rapidly acquire information about their environments, (2) quickly adapt their behaviours and structures to changing circumstances, (3) communicate easily and thoroughly with others, and (4) broadly mobilize networks of expertise and material support.[304, 305] At the individual level, resilience is the process of negotiating, managing and adapting to significant sources of stress or trauma. Assets and resources within the individual, their life and environment facilitate this capacity for adaptation and 'bouncing back' in the face of adversity.[306, 307]

RESPONDER STATUS

See TREATMENT BENEFIT.

RESPONSE SHIFT

A change in the meaning of one's self-evaluation of a target construct as a result of: (a) a change in the respondent's internal standards of measurement (scale recalibration, in psychometric terms); (b) a change in the respondent's values (i.e. the importance of component domains constituting the target construct); or (c) a redefinition of the target construct (i.e. reconceptualization).[39]

> 1.RECALIBRATION: A change in the values or rating assigned to a health state based on a person changing their perception of the value rather than experiencing a true change.[39]
>
> 2. REPRIORITIZATION: A type of response shift where people change what is important to them when evaluating their quality of life.[308, 309]
>
> 3. RECONCEPTUALIZATION: A component of response shift in which there is a change in the meaning of one's self-evaluation of a target construct as a result of a redefinition of the target construct (i.e. reconceptualization); this can be detected statistically using Structural Equation Modeling; alternately personalized measures of quality of life can also detect this when people nominate different areas of their life affected by disease over time.[39]

RESPONSIVENESS

See CHANGE.

RETROSPECTIVE

Examining events that occurred in the past over a specified period of time. This type of observation may be applied to case-control studies and certain types of cohort studies; for cohort studies, the term historical cohort is preferred to retrospective cohort study.[17]

RISK FACTOR

Any social (e.g. domestic violence), economic (e.g. poverty), biological (e.g. inheriting a breast cancer gene), behavioural (e.g. smoking) or environmental (e.g. poor housing, pollution) factor that is associated with or can cause an increased risk of a particular disease, injury or physical or mental illness.[12]

S

SCALE

A term often used (erroneously) to refer to a measure or questionnaire when it should only be used to describe the response categories on an item.[51] See also MEASUREMENT SCALE.

SCOPING REVIEW

One method amongst many that might be used to review literature. Scoping reviews share some similarities with systematic reviews but differ in several important ways. The question is more exploratory in nature as the aim is usually to examine the extent, range, and nature of research activity in a particular field without necessarily abstracting data or attempting to assess its quality. Scoping reviews produce a profile of the existing literature in a topic area, which may point to areas where a systematic review would be helpful or identify areas in the literature where gaps exist. The scoping process is iterative and is used to estimate the size of the literature in question, and the estimated costs of searching it. There is a greater need for a scoping review when the topic to be searched is interdisciplinary.[310, 311]

SCREENING

The use of tests to help diagnose disease or their precursor conditions, in the earlier phase of their natural history or at the less severe spectrum than usual. The assumption of screening is that the people being screened are presumed normal in that they have no symptoms or overt manifestations of disease. Screening differs from case finding, diagnosis among the symptomatic, even though the same test may be used. Screening should be reserved for conditions where there is an effective intervention when earlier intervention improves outcome. If the screening test can recognize earlier disease the test is available, affordable and acceptable, the disease is a health priority and the benefits of screening exceed the cost.[5] Screening for many cancers is recommended but screening for some fatal neurological conditions with no effective treatment is debated and is a matter of personal choice.[312]

SECONDARY PREVENTION

See PREVENTION.

SECOND LIFE

Second Life, created by San Francisco based company Linden Labs in 2003, is an online virtual reality world where users, called residents, create their own virtual selves, called avatars, and interact within a simulated 3-D environment, literally living a virtual "Second Life". It has a number of health-related applications including education, health awareness, support groups, and even recruitment of real subjects into research projects. It is an interesting environment for people with disabilities allowing them to have experiences not available to them in the "real" world. There is evidence that behaviours learned in the virtual world transfer into the "real" world.[313]

SELF-EFFICACY

Perceived self-efficacy refers to beliefs that individuals hold about their capability to carry out action in a way that will influence the events that affect their lives. Self-efficacy beliefs determine how people feel, think, motivate themselves and behave.[32, 314]

SELF-MANAGEMENT

The individual's ability to manage the symptoms, treatment, physical and psychosocial consequences and lifestyle changes inherent in living with a chronic condition. Self-management includes four activities: (i) engaging in activities that promote health and build physiological reserve, such as exercise, proper nutrition, social activation, and sleep; (ii) interaction with health care providers and systems and adherence to recommended treatment protocols; (iii) regular monitoring of physical and emotional status and making appropriate adjustments on the basis of symptoms and signs; and (iv) managing the impact of the illness on ability to function in important roles, on emotions and self-esteem, and on relations with others. The best known self-management program is the Stanford Self-Management Program from the USA[315], the Expert Patient Programme from the UK[316], and the Flinders from Australia.[317] In all cases, these programs aim to promote patients' empowerment to cope with diseases while achieving an optimal level of quality of life.[315-320]

SELF-RATED HEALTH

How a person would rate his or her health based on their own perception, experience, and frame of reference; common response options are: Excellent, Very good, Good, Fair, Poor (EVGGFP); or a 0 to 100 or 0 to 10 visual analogue scale (VAS).[321-323] See also GENERAL HEALTH PERCEPTION

SENSITIVITY

Probability that a diagnostic technique will detect a particular disease or condition when it does indeed exist in a patient; it is calculated as the proportion of people with the with a disorder according to a gold standard or reference test who score in the positive (or affected) range on a different or index test; also referred to as the proportion of true positives and 1-sensitivity is the proportion of false positives.[76] See also SPECIFICITY.

SENSITIVITY ANALYSIS

Mathematical calculation that isolate factors involved in a decision analysis or economic analysis to indicate the degree of influence each factor has on the outcome of the entire analysis. It measures the uncertainty of the probability distributions.[180]

SEX

Refers to the biological characteristics such as anatomy (e.g. body size and shape) and physiology (e.g. hormonal activity or functioning of organs) that distinguish males and females.[39]

SIGN

An objective indication of some medical fact or characteristics that may be detected through a physical examination of a patient; swelling of a joint is a sign of inflammation.[120]

SINGLE ITEM MEASURE

One question that has been shown to accurately assess a construct.[324, 325]

SINGLE SUBJECT (CASE) DESIGN

Type of experimental study of a single subject ideally suited for studying behavior change when variability across individuals is large and variability within the person is the target of study.[326]

SNOWBALL SAMPLING

A type of respondent-driven sampling suitable for selecting members of "hidden" populations into studies; sometimes used to obtain data from hard to approach populations such as illicit drug users, or members of specific groups such as health professionals. The aim is to use each person to identify people like themselves. A closely related method is network sampling where a person is asked to identify people within their social network who may or may not share similar characteristics. These types of non-random sampling increase power but cannot be used to estimate population parameters as the extent to which the sample represents the population is inestimable.[65]

SOCIAL DESIRABILITY BIAS

The need for subjects to respond in socially sanctioned ways.[327] This bias can arise from wording of questions in such a way that it is uncomfortable for people to tell the truth. Therefore, when writing questions on issues that are subject to social desirability it is important to word the item so that people can admit to doing something they perceive they should not or *vice versa*. This bias can also arise owing to a personality trait where people are more likely to provide an answer based on what they perceive as more acceptable because they want to appear to be a "good" person. The first source of bias can be minimized by good question design; the second source of bias probably needs a measure of this tendency to aid in the interpretation of responses.[90, 327, 328]

SOCIAL DETERMINANTS OF HEALTH

The circumstances, in which people are born, grow up, live, work and age, and the systems put in place to deal with illness. These circumstances are in turn shaped by a wider set of forces: economics, social policies, and politics.[165]

SOCIAL ENVIRONMENT

The aggregate of social and cultural institutions, norms, patterns, beliefs, and processes that influence the life of an individual or community. It includes interactions with family, friends, coworkers and others in the community, as well as cultural attitudes, norms, and expectations. It encompasses social relationships and policies in settings such as schools, neighbourhoods, workplaces, businesses, places of worship, health care settings, recreation facilities, and other public places. It includes the social aspects of health-related behaviours (e.g., tobacco use, substance use, physical activity) in the community. It also encompasses social institutions like law enforcement (e.g., the presence or lack of community policing), and governmental as well as non-governmental organizations.[256]

SOCIAL EPIDEMIOLOGY

The study of health and illness in populations which is informed by social, psychological, economic and public policy information, and uses that information in defining and proposing solutions for public health problem.[105]

SOCIAL INTEGRATION

The extent to which an individual participates in a broad range of social relationships. People who are more socially integrated live longer and experience other health benefits through having more diverse self-concepts (spouse, parent, friend, worker, member of a group, etc.), a more diverse resource pool to call upon when under stress, and better quality and quantity of social interactions. Diversity acts as a buffer for stressful events and quality social interactions decrease negative affects and increase positive effects.[69]

SOCIAL INTEGRATED COMMUNITIES

The extent to which communities offer their members opportunities to increase their personal and family resources through increased opportunity for active involvement in formal.[69]

SOCIAL FUNCTION

The actions and tasks required for basic and complex interactions with people in a contextually and socially appropriate manner; social function is related to social support as someone who is socially functional will likely have a strong social support system in place that could be used as a coping mechanism.[7]

SOCIAL GRADIENT IN HEALTH

Runs from top to bottom of the socioeconomic spectrum where the poorest of the poor, around the world, have the worst health. This is a global phenomenon, seen in low, middle and high income countries. Within countries, the evidence shows that in general the lower an individual's socioeconomic position the worse their health.[165]

SOCIAL PARTICIPATION

A person's involvement in activities that provide interaction with others in society or the community[329]; a means of carrying out one's life habits in one's environment (e.g., school, work place, neighbourhood.[330]

SOCIAL SUPPORT

An expression of a personal relationship that is characterized by a sense of attachment, intimacy, mutuality, and solidarity. Social support is not a variable but a process which means that it is not a commodity or resource that can be dispensed by one party to another. Social support occurs when there is an environment that is supportive, non-threatening, and permits creativity (in the broadest sense of the word). Social support can take the form of emotional support, instrumental or tangible, practical support in the form of assistance or material aid, informational support, companionship, or validation of individuals behaviours or feelings with respect to social norms.[69]

SORROW

A natural response to losses brought on by illness or injury; it is sometimes differentiated from bereavement in that the response is to living loss. Episodes of sadness and grief-related feelings occur, and in between these episodes the person functions normally.[331]

SPEARMAN RANK ORDER CORRELATION

See CORRELATION COEFFICIENT.

SPECIFICITY

The proportion of people previously identified as free of a particular disorder who score in the negative (unaffected) range on a new diagnostic test; also referred to as the rate of true negatives; 1-specificity is the rate of false negatives; in the context of screening, a higher rate of false negatives (people are told they may have a disease when they do not) is more acceptable than a high rate of false positives (people who are told they are disease free when they actually have the disease)[76]. See also SENSITIVITY.

STANDARD GAMBLE

A classical approach derived from the fundamental axioms of utility theory used to measure utility. Respondents are asked to choose between two possible outcomes of a hypothetical situation: Choice A is an uncertain choice and contains two possible health state outcomes each with a probability of occurring. Choice B is a certain choice with 100% probability of occurring. For example, a respondent is asked to imagine that he has chronic renal failure and is being treated in a dialysis unit. Choice A is to gamble on a kidney transplant that has a probability p of bringing about a state of complete health, but also has a probability $1-p$ of immediate death from surgery. Choice B is to remain on dialysis for the rest of his life with complete certainty.[181]

STANDARD DEVIATION

A measure of a spread of a given set of numbers calculated as the root mean squared deviation of these values from their mean.[332]

STANDARD ERROR

The variability of the mean of the sample as an estimate of the true value of the mean for the population. It is equal to the standard deviation divided by the square root of the sample size. It can be used to describe an interval within which we can say with a given level of certainty that the true population mean lies. The standard error is used for inference and is not a descriptive statistic and hence it should not be reported when the observed data obtained on the sample is being described, the standard deviation should be reported as the descriptive statistic for observed data.[239] In statistical modeling, it is the standard deviation of the estimated parameter.

STANDARD ERROR OF MEASUREMENT (SEM)

A measure of how apart the values are with repeated measurements. It is calculated as the square root of the error variance from in the intraclass correlation coefficient (ICC) formula.[2]

STANDARDIZED RESPONSE MEAN

A measure of effect size calculated by dividing the mean change by the standard deviation of the change scores.[50]

STATISTICALLY SIGNIFICANT

Conclusion based on a statistical test that the observed result is unlikely to have occurred by chance alone.[275]

STEPPED WEDGE

A type of randomised trial design that involves sequential implementation of an intervention to participants (individuals or clusters) over a number of time periods. By the end of the study, all participants will have received the intervention. A critical feature is randomization of the order in which participants receive the intervention (see Figure). The design is particularly relevant where it is predicted that the intervention will do more good than harm (making a parallel design, in which certain participants do not receive the intervention, unethical) and/or when there are issues of resources and training such that not all participants can enter the intervention at the same time. Data analysis focuses on modelling the effect of time on the effectiveness of an intervention. This is one of the designs suitable for implementation science or knowledge translation.[333, 334]

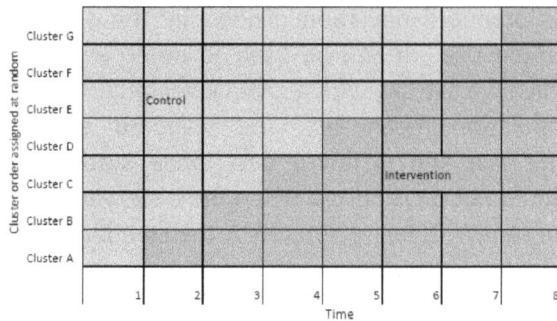

STRUCTURAL EQUATION MODELING (SEM)

Family of related multivariate sophisticated statistical procedures for testing how well theoretical models conform to the data; SEM consists of two basic elements: a measurement model, analysed by factor analysis, and a structural model, by path analysis. SEM uses latent variables to represent the constructs of interest recognizing that complex constructs are not adequately represented by any one single measure and the commonality between related measures is a better representation.[54, 335]

STRUCTURAL VALIDITY

The degree to which the scores of an instrument are an adequate reflection of the dimensionality of the construct to be measured.[46]

STRUCTURED REVIEW

A form of review that is structured in terms of defining explicit search, selection, data extraction, and appraisal criteria but done by primarily by one reviewer.[336, 337] See also SYSTEMATIC REVIEWS.

SUBSCALE

Many measurement instruments are multidimensional and are designed to measure more than one construct or more than one domain of a single construct. In such instances subscales can be constructed in which the various items from a scale are grouped into subscales. Although a subscale could consist of a single item, in most cases subscales consist of multiple individual items that have been combined into a composite score. The values on these different subscales produce a profile for an individual.[338]

SUPERIORITY STUDY OR TRIAL

A randomized controlled trial with the aim of showing that an experimental treatment is statistically and clinically superior to the active control treatment; used when a placebo would be unethical or otherwise inappropriate. The null hypothesis is that the experimental group is not different from the control group and the alternative hypothesis is that the experimental treatment is superior.[232] See also NON-INFERIORITY TRIAL.

SURVIVOR

An individual who has survived a health condition that is often fatal; used in the context of a stroke survivor or a cancer survivor. In terms of a cancer survivor, there is a debate as to when a person becomes a survivor; for some a person is a survivor from the time of cancer diagnosis through the balance of his or her life; for others, a person is not a survivor until the end of primary treatment.[52]

SURVIVORSHIP CARE

A distinct phase of care for cancer survivors that includes four components: (1) prevention and detection of new cancers and recurrent cancer; (2) surveillance for cancer spread, recurrence, or second cancers; (3) intervention for consequences of cancer and its treatment; and (4) coordination between specialists and primary care providers to ensure that all of the survivor's health needs are met.[52]

SURVIVORSHIP RESEARCH

Research encompasses the physical, psychosocial, and economic sequelae of cancer diagnosis and its treatment among both pediatric and adult survivors of cancer. It also includes within its domain issues related to health care delivery, access, and follow-up care, as they relate to survivors.[52]

SYMPTOM

A perception, belief or abnormal feeling held or noticed by the patient that could indicate the presence of a disease or an abnormality. Symptoms can only be measured by patient-reported outcomes (PRO). Symptoms have the dimensions of intensity, frequency, duration, nature, impact, and bother.[223, 255]

SYNDROME

A group of signs and symptoms that occur together and characterize a particular abnormality.[92]

SYNTHESIS

Synthesis, in this context, means the contextualization and integration of research findings of individual research studies within the larger body of knowledge on the topic. A synthesis must be reproducible and transparent in its methods, using quantitative and/or qualitative methods. It could take the form of a systematic review, follow the methods developed by the Cochrane Collaboration, result from a consensus conference or expert panel or synthesize qualitative or quantitative results. Realist syntheses, narrative syntheses, meta-analyses, meta-syntheses and practice guidelines are all forms of synthesis.[108]

SYSTEMATIC REVIEW

Empirical evidence, that meets pre-defined eligibility criteria, collated to answer a specific research question. This entails using an explicit and systematic methodology that is chosen in order to minimize bias therefore providing findings that are reliable and in which conclusions and decisions can be made. The key characteristics of a systematic review include: (1) objectives that are clear with pre-defined eligibility criteria; (2) methodology that is explicit and can be reproduced; (3) a search of studies that is thorough and systematic that will identify all studies meeting the pre-defined eligibility criteria; (4) an assessment of the validity of the findings of the included studies (e.g. assess risk bias); and (5) a systematic presentation, and synthesis, of the characteristics and findings of the included studies. Many systematic reviews will also include meta-analyses.[336, 337, 339] See also META-ANALYSIS.

T

TELECARE

A combination of equipment, monitoring and response that can help individuals to remain independent at home. Common examples include detectors for falls, fire or gas and trigger a warning to a response centre, vital sign monitors to provide early warning of deterioration, prompting a response from family or professionals.[12]

TELEHEALTH

Delivery of health-related services and information via telecommunications technologies.[12]

TELEMEDICINE

The practice of medical care using interactive audio visual and data communications, this includes the delivery of medical care, diagnosis, consultation, and treatment, as well as health education and the transfer of medical information.[12]

TERTIARY PREVENTION

See PREVENTION.

TEST-RETEST RELIABILITY

A way of estimating the reliability of a scale in which individuals are administered the same scale on two different occasions and then the two scores are assessed for consistency. This method of evaluating reliability is appropriate only if the phenomenon that the scale measures is known to be stable over the interval between assessments. If the phenomenon being measured fluctuates substantially over time, then the test-retest paradigm may significantly underestimate reliability. In using test-retest reliability, the investigator needs to take into account the possibility of practice effects, which can artificially inflate the estimate of reliability.[18, 338]

THEN-TEST

A design based method for evaluating changes in internal standards, a component of response shift. In the context of a longitudinal observational study or clinical trial, patients are asked to fill out a questionnaire on some aspect of their health or quality of life at each visit (e.g. pre and post). At a follow-up assessment, patients are asked to complete the post version and also to provide a renewed judgement of their earlier assessment based on their current standards. As the two ratings, the post and the renewed pre are completed using the same internal standards, the difference between the original pre and the renewed pre are considered a measure of response shift.[308]

THEORY

An organized, heuristic, coherent, and systematic articulation of a set of statements related to significant questions that are communicated in a meaningful whole. It describes observations, summarizes current evidence, proposes, explanations, and yields testable hypotheses. It is a symbolic depiction of aspects of reality that are discovered or invented for describing, explaining, predicting, and controlling a phenomenon. Simply spoken, it is akin to a road map, and as such it is context specific.[221, 222]

TIME-TRADE-OFF (TTO)

A method of measuring health-state preferences in which patients are asked to trade off life years in a state of less-than-perfect health for a shorter life span in a state of perfect health. The ratio of the number of years of perfect health that is equivalent to longer life span in less-than-perfect health provides a measure of the preference for that health state.[180]

TOOL

See INSTRUMENT.

TRANSDISCIPLINARITY

The philosophical concept of scholarly inquiry that ignores conventional boundaries among ways of thinking about and solving problems. It is based on recognition of the inherent complexity of many problems confronting humans and has evolved a conceptual framework that embraces and seeks to mobilize all pertinent scientific and scholarly disciplines: physical, biological, social and behavioural sciences, ethics, moral philosophy, communication sciences, economics, politics, and the humanities. Many problems in public health require an inherently transdisciplinary approach. The social, demographic, and human health problems associated with global environmental change demand the greatest degree of transdisciplinarity. The advantage of this approach is that "new science" is created, ways of thinking and solving problems that do not currently exist but develop out of the collective wisdom.

TRANSFORMATIVE LEARNING

An adult learning theory that is used to understand the processes by which adults change or transform how they think about their lives as they encounter new challenges, such as being diagnosed with and living with a chronic or new health condition. It is a dynamic process entailing growth and learning as new experiences occur, and results in a restructuring of the illness experience and restructuring of self, leading to new rules, behaviors, feelings, beliefs, perspectives, and identity. Transformative learning has many similarities with response shift as well as differences. Response shift focuses on theory development, quantitative and qualitative methods for detection, and applications for clinical practice and research. Transformative learning focuses on adaptation and personal growth in the context of living with a health conditions. Response shift phenomena are not necessarily within the awareness of the individual, whereas transformative learning is clearly defined in terms of a critical reflection process for developing a new personal reality.[340]

TRANSLATABILITY ASSESSMENT

The evaluation of the extent to which a measure can be meaningfully translated into another language where "meaningful" implies a translation that is conceptually equivalent to the source text and culturally and linguistically appropriate in the target country. TA is done prior to translation to identify translation difficulties. When these are identified a number of solutions are available: (a) changing the original wording of the item in the source language; or (b) retaining the original wording in the source language and providing alternative wording on which potential translations in the target language may be based.[2, 341]

TREATMENT BENEFIT

A favorable effect on a meaningful aspect of how a patient feels or functions in their life, or on survival where meaningful refers to the effect on an aspect of health affected by the disease that is manifested by how the patient feels or functions, the patient cares about and prefers that it is prevented, improved, or does not become worse. This favourable effect should occur in the patient's typical life and not just be change in performance of specific task in a testing situation, a task that the patient is unlikely to do or wish to do in their usual life. Investigators proposing such a test need to demonstrate its meaning for patients lives even in the absence of face validity.[55, 342] The criteria to define treatment benefit can be used define responder status a clinical trial.

TYPE I ERROR

The erroneous conclusion that two treatments differ, when in reality they do not.[17]

TYPE II ERROR

Failing to detect a difference between treatments when in reality one truly exists.[17]

U

UNIVERSAL COVERAGE

An approach to health care funding ensuring that all people have access to needed health services – prevention, promotion, treatment and rehabilitation – without facing financial ruin because of the need to pay for them. Synonyms: universal health coverage, social health protection.[343]

UTILITY

Individual's or society's preference for any particular set of health outcomes.[181]

UTILITY SCALE

Scale reflecting strength of preferences for uncertain outcomes.[181]

UTILITY THEORY

It is a set of assumptions about how to quantify people's choices and decisions along a continuum from preference to indifference.[344]

V

VALIDITY

Relative lack of systematic error. In the context of measuring constructs that have no gold standard or true value, the term validity has evolved to indicate what conclusions can be drawn about a person based on a test result. Validity is not a property of the test or assessment as such, but rather of the meaning of the test scores. In short, validity is an overall assessment of the degree to which evidence and theory support the interpretation of scores entailed by proposed uses of the instrument. Simply put, it is the degree to which an assessment measures what it is supposed to measure.[4, 345]

VALUATION

Process used to elicit persons' values or preferences for a health state; several methods are described in the literature such as standard gamble, time trade off, rating scale, and willingness-to-pay.[346]

VALUE

The foundation of an individual's thoughts, feelings, beliefs and attitudes.[12] Four broad groups of values have been identified: (i) ethical value, those related to equality, freedom, honesty, and responsibility; (ii) psychological value in terms of cognitive or emotional goodness; (iii) social value related to improvements in the lives of individuals or society as a whole or anything that allows an individual to fulfill the roles expected by society; and (iv) economic value such as ability to earn, manage and spend money efficiently.[347-349]

VALUE SCALE

Scale of preferences for certain or sure outcomes.[181]

VERBAL RATING SCALE (VRS)

Ordered categorical scale, with each response option consisting of adjectives. For different levels of PI, "no pain," "mild pain," "moderate pain," "severe pain," "extreme pain," and the "most intense pain imaginable" form a six category VRS scale (VRS-6). VRS scales are commonly of lengths four to seven. The adjectives are scored by assigning numbers (0-6) to each response option. The scale also may be called VPS (Verbal Pain Scale), VDS (Verbal Descriptor Scale), or SDS (Simple Descriptor Scale).[235]

VISUAL ANALOG SCALE (VAS)

A visual analogue scale (VAS) is a response format intended to record numerical ratings on a continuum. A classic VAS consists of a line about 10 or 20 cm long with the ends labelled to indicate what the most extreme values represent. The line can be horizontal or vertical. An example would be an item to measure post-surgical pain, with the ends labelled "no pain" and "worse imaginable pain". The respondent is instructed to place a tick mark or cross the point on this line that represents their experience of pain. When completed by pencil and paper, a scorer needs to use a ruler to obtain the VAS score. VAS-like formats, that include markings like a thermometer, eliminate the need for hand scoring. The EQ-5D health state item is an example of a thermometer-style VAS.[149, 149, 235, 350, 350]

W

WEB-BASED INTERVENTION

A self-guided intervention program that is executed by means of a prescriptive online program operated through a website and used by consumers seeking health- or mental-health related assistance. The intervention program itself attempts to create positive change and or improve/enhance knowledge, awareness, and understanding via the provision of sound health-related material and use of interactive web-based components.[351]

WEIGHT-RELATED QUALITY OF LIFE

The effect of excess weight on the ability to lead a fulfilling life.[352, 353]

WELLNESS

The optimal state of health of individuals and groups. There are two focal concerns: the realization of the fullest potential of an individual physically, psychologically, socially, spiritually and economically, and the fulfilment of one's role expectations in the family, community, place of worship, workplace and other settings.[32]

WELL-BEING

A construct related to what it means to be self-actualized, a distinct individual, fully functioning, and optimally developed; well-being has roots in concepts of happiness, life satisfaction and positive affect. Its core dimensions are considered to encompass purpose in life, personal growth, positive relations with others, environmental mastery, self-acceptance, and autonomy.[123, 354]

WILLINGNESS-TO-PAY

In the context of health outcomes, it is the maximum amount a person would be willing to pay in order to avoid a negative outcome or receive a positive outcome; it is often contrasted with the actual cost of the something known to produce the desired outcome such as a drug, test or procedure.

WILSON-CLEARY MODEL

A conceptual and model, taxonomy of patient outcomes, that categorizes patient outcomes according to the underlying health concepts they represent and proposes specific causal relationships between different health concepts, thereby integrating the biomedical model and quality of life. The components of health-related quality of life are linked under the rubrics of biological and physiological variables, symptoms, function, health perception, and quality of life, recognizing the influence of personal factors (symptom amplification, motivation, personality, values and preferences), environmental factors (psychological, social and economic supports, and non-medical factors). This model is closely linked to the biopsychosocial model of the WHO's ICF where biological variables and symptoms would be classified as impairments, and function includes activity and participation domains.[118, 355]

WORLD HEALTH ORGANIZATION (WHO)

An agency of the United Nations (UN) located in Geneva, Switzerland, with a primary role to direct and coordinate international health. Established in 1948, it works in the areas of health systems, promoting health through the life-course, noncommunicable diseases, communicable diseases, preparedness, surveillance and response. See also HEALTH

Y

YEA-SAYING

Tendency of respondents to agree rather than disagree with statements as a whole or with what are perceived to be socially desirable responses to the question, also called acquiescence bias.[152] See also ACQUIESCENCE BIAS

Z

Z-SCORE

A standard score obtained by transforming a variable to have a mean of zero and a standard deviation of one. The score is calculated by subtracting off the population mean from the test subject's observed score and dividing by the standard deviation of the normative population.[2, 5]

REFERENCE LIST

1. Landau SI. Dictionaries: The Art and Craft of Lexicography. 2nd ed. Press Syndicate of the University of Cambridge; 2001.

2. de Vet HC, Terwee CB, Mokkink LB, Knol DL. Measurement in Medicine. Cambridge University Press; 2011.

3. Everitt BS. Cambridge Dictionary of Statistics. 3 ed. United Kingdom: Cambridge University Press; 2006.

4. Streiner DL, Norman GR. Health Measurement Scale: a practical guide to their development and use. Fourth ed. Oxford; 2008.

5. Porta M. A Dictionary of Epidemiology. 5th ed. Oxford University Press; 2008.

6. Sackett DL. Bias in analytic research. J Chronic Dis 1979;32(1-2):51-63.

7. WHO. International Classification of Functioning, Disability and Health. Second revision. ed. Geneva: 2001.

8. Katz S, Ford AB, Moskowitz RW, Jackson BA, Jaffe MW. Studies of illness in the aged. the Index of ADL: A standardized measure of biological and psychosocial function. JAMA 1963;185:914-919.

9. Weiss DJ, Kingsbury GG. Application of computerized adaptive testing to educational problems. Journal of Educational Measurement 1984;21:361-375.

10. World Health Organization. Adherence to Long-Term Therapies- Evidence to Action. 2003.

11. American Cancer Society. American Cancer Society. http://www.cancer.org/ . 2011.

12. NHS Care Records Service- Single Assessment Process. Glossary of Health, Social Care and Information Technology. 2011.

13. VandenBos GR. APA Dictionary of Psychology. Washington DC: American Psychological Association; 2007.

14. Oxford Dictionaries. The Oxford Dictionary. Oxford University Press; 2010.

15. Graciano WG, Torbin RM. Agreeableness. In: Leary MR, Hoyle RH, editors. Handbook of Individual Differences in Social Behavior. New York: Guilford Press; 2009:46-61.

16. Fleiss J. Statistical Methods for Rates and Proportions. 2nd ed. New York: John Wiley & Sons; 1981.

17. Gordis L. Epidemiology. 3rd ed. Philadelphia, PA: Elsevier Saunders; 2004.

18. de Vet HC, Terwee CB, Mokkink LB. Measurement in Medicine: A Practical Guide. New York: Cambridge University Press; 2011.

19. Health Insurance Portability and Accountability Act. HIPAA Glossary. http://healthcare.partners.org/phsirb/hipaaglos.htm#g3), 1996.

20. Marin RS. Apathy: a neuropsychiatric syndrome. J Neuropsychiatry Clin Neurosci 1991;3(3):243-254.

21. Robert P, Onyike CU, Leentjens AF et al. Proposed diagnostic criteria for apathy in Alzheimer's disease and other neuropsychiatric disorders. Eur Psychiatry 2009;24(2):98-104.

22. Starkstein S. Apathy and Withdrawal. Int Psychogeriatr 2000;12:135-137.

23. Lourenco CB. Apathy in Stroke: Conceptualization, Measurement, and Impact. McGill University; 2014.

24. Rapkin BD, Schwartz CE. Toward a theoretical model of quality-of-life appraisal: Implications of findings from studies of response shift. Health Qual Life Outcomes 2004;2:14.

25. Stanford Encyclopedia of Philosophy. Stanford California: 2010.

26. Guillemin F, Bombardier C, Beaton D. Cross-cultural adaptation of health-related quality of life measures: literature review and proposed guidelines. J Clin Epidemiol 1993;46(12):1417-1432.

27. Cook KF, Victorson DE, Cella D, Schalet BD, Miller D. Creating meaningful cut-scores for Neuro-QOL measures of fatigue, physical functioning, and sleep disturbance using standard setting with patients and providers. Qual Life Res 2015;24(3):575-589.

28. UCLA: Institute for Digital Research and Education. Regression with SAS: Simple and Multiple Regression. http://www.ats.ucla.edu/stat/sas/webbooks/reg/chapter1/sasreg1.htm), 2015.

29. Simon Day. Dictionary for Clinical Trials. Second Edition ed. Welwyn Garden City: Roche Products Limited; 2007.

30. US National Library of Medicine: National Institutes of Health. http://www.nlm.nih.gov/ . 2012.

31. Eton DT, Ramalho de OD, Egginton JS et al. Building a measurement framework of burden of treatment in complex patients with chronic conditions: a qualitative study. Patient Relat Outcome Meas 2012;3:39-49.

32. WHO Glossary. http://www.who.int/health-systems-performance/docs/glossary.htm . 2000.

33. Smith BJ, Tang KC, Nutbeam D. WHO Health Promotion Glossary: new terms. Health Promotion International 2006;21(4):340-345.

34. WHO. Glossary of globalization, trade and health terms. http://www.who.int/trade/glossary/en/ . 2011.

35. Schlesselman JJ, Stolley PD. Case-Control Studies. Design, Conduct, Analysis. Monographs in Epidemiology and Biostatistics. New York, Oxford: Oxford University Press; 1982:7-26.

36. Mayo NE, Goldberg MS. When is a case-control study a case-control study? J Rehabil Med 2009;41(4):217-222.

37. Mayo NE, Goldberg MS. When is a case-control study not a case-control study? J Rehabil Med 2009;41(4):209-216.

38. Schwandt TA. Qualitative Inquiry: A Dictionary of Terms. SAGE Publications Inc; 1997.

39. Sprangers MA, Schwartz CE. Integrating response shift into health-related quality of life research: a theoretical model. Soc Sci Med 1999;48(11):1507-1515.

40. Fayers PM, Hand DJ. Factor analysis, causal indicators and quality of life. Qual Life Res 1997;6(2):139-150.

41. Fayers P, Machin D. Quality of Life: The Assessment, Analysis, and Interpretation of Patient-reported Outcomes. 2 ed. Wiley; 2007.

42. Rothman KJ. Causes. Am J Epidemiol 1976;104(6):587-592.

43. Fayers PM. Causal Variables in Quality of Life Measurement. Open University Press; 1997.

44. Beaton DE. Understanding the relevance of measured change through studies of responsiveness. Spine (Phila Pa 1976) 2000;25(24):3192-3199.

45. Jaeschke R, Singer J, Guyatt GH. Measurement of health status. Ascertaining the minimal clinically important difference. Controlled Clinical Trials 1989;10:407-415.

46. Mokkink LB, Terwee CB, Patrick DL et al. The COSMIN study reached international consensus on taxonomy, terminology, and definitions of measurement properties for health-related patient-reported outcomes. J Clin Epidemiol 2010;63(7):737-745.

47. Norman GR, Sloan JA, Wyrwich KW. Interpretation of changes in health-related quality of life: the remarkable universality of half a standard deviation. Med Care 2003;41(5):582-592.

48. Hrobjartsson A, Gotzsche PC. Is the placebo powerless? An analysis of clinical trials comparing placebo with no treatment. N Engl J Med 2001;344(21):1594-1602.

49. Terwee CB, Dekker FW, Wiersinga WM, Prummel MF, Bossuyt PM. On assessing responsiveness of health-related quality of life instruments: guidelines for instrument evaluation. Qual Life Res 2003;12(4):349-362.

50. Liang MH, Larson MG, Cullen KE, Schwartz JA. Comparative measurement efficiency and sensitivity of five health status

instruments for arthritis research. Arthritis & Rheumatism 1985;28(5):542-547.

51. Sloan JA, Aaronson N, Cappelleri JC, Fairclough DL, Varricchio C. Assessing the clinical significance of single items relative to summated scores. Mayo Clin Proc 2002;77(5):479-487.

52. From Cancer patient to Cancer Survivor: Lost in Translation. Glossary of Common Cancer Terms. www.iom.edu . 2006.

53. Wagner EH, Austin BT, Von KM. Organizing care for patients with chronic illness. Milbank Q 1996;74(4):511-544.

54. Kilne RB. Principles and Practices of Structural Equation Modeling. Second ed. New York: Guilford Press; 2005.

55. Federal Drug Administration (FDA). Patient Reported Outcome Measures: Use in Medical Production Development to Support Labeling Claims. 2009.

56. Mayo NE. Randomized Trials and Other Parallel Comparisons of Treatment. In: Bailar JC, Hoaglin DC, editors. Medical Uses of Statistics. 3rd ed. Hoboken, New Jersey: A John Wiley & Sons, Inc & The New England Journal of Medicine; 2009:51-89.

57. Willke RJ, Burke LB, Erickson P. Measuring treatment impact: a review of patient-reported outcomes and other efficacy endpoints in approved product labels. Control Clin Trials 2004;25(6):535-552.

58. Feinstein AR. Clinimetrics. New Haven and London: 1987.

59. Klar N, Donner A. Current and future challenges in the design and analysis of cluster randomization trials. Stat Med 2001;20(24):3729-3740.

60. The Cochrane Collaborators. Cochrane Hanbook for Systematic Reviews of Interventions. Higgins JPT, Green S, editors. www.cochrane-handbook.org . 2011.

61. Willis G, Roston P, Bercini D. The use of verbal report methods in the development and testing of survey questionnaires. Applied Cognitive Psychology 1991;5:251-267.

62. Kipling R. The Elephant's Child. Just So Stories For Little Children. eBooks@Adelaide; 1902.

63. Blair J, Conrad FG. Sample Size for Cognitive Interview Pretesting. Public Opinion Quarterly 2011;75(4):636-658.

64. Relton C, Torgerson D, O'Cathain A, Nicholl J. Rethinking pragmatic randomised controlled trials: introducing the "cohort multiple randomised controlled trial" design. BMJ 2010;340:c1066.

65. Last JM. A Dictionary of Epidemiology. Fourth ed. Oxford University Press; 2001.

66. Allison PD. Missing Data. Thousand Oaks, California: Sage Publications, Inc.; 2002.

67. Mukherjee B, Ou HT, Wang F, Erickson SR. A new comorbidity index: the health-related quality of life comorbidity index. J Clin Epidemiol 2011;64(3):309-319.

68. Deyo RA, Cherkin DC, Ciol MA. Adapting a clinical comorbidity index for use with ICD-9-CM administrative databases. Journal of Clinical Epidemiology 1992;45:613-619.

69. Cohen S, Underwood LG, Gottlieb BH. Social Support Measurement and Intervention: A Guide for Health and Social Scientists. New York: Oxford University Press; 2001.

70. Institute of Medicine. Institute of Medicine. http://www.iom.edu/ . 2011.

71. Bagiella E. Clinical trials in rehabilitation: single or multiple outcomes? Arch Phys Med Rehabil 2009;90(11 Suppl):S17-S21.

72. Tilley BC, Marler J, Geller NL et al. Use of a global test for multiple outcomes in stroke trials with application to the National Institute of Neurological Disorders and Stroke t-PA Stroke Trial. Stroke 1996;27(11):2136-2142.

73. OECD Glossary of Statistical terms. http://stats.oecd.org/glossary/), 2012.

74. Trochim WM, Linton R. Conceptualization for planning and evaluation. Evaluation and program planning 1986;9(4):289-308.

75. Jenkinson C, Gray A, Doll H, Lawrence K, Keoghane S, Layte R. Evaluation of index and profile measures of health status in a randomized controlled trial. Comparison of the Medical Outcomes Study 36-Item Short Form Health Survey, EuroQol, and disease specific measures. Med Care 1997;35(11):1109-1118.

76. Center for Evidence-Based Center - KT Clearinghouse. Glossary of Evidence-Based Medicine. http://ktclearinghouse.ca/cebm/glossary/#glossary_a . 2011.

77. de Vet HC, Ader HJ, Terwee CB, Pouwer F. Are factor analytical techniques used appropriately in the validation of health status questionnaires? A systematic review on the quality of factor analysis of the SF-36. Qual Life Res 2005;14(5):1203-1218.

78. Floyd FJ, Widaman KF. Factor analysis in the development and refinement of clinical assessment instruments. Psychological Assessment 1995;7:286-299.

79. Fairclough DL. Summary measures and statistics for comparison of quality of life in a clinical trial of cancer therapy. Stat Med 1997;16(11):1197-1209.

80. Ryan M, Farrar S. Eliciting preferences for health care using conjoint analysis. BMJ 2000;320:1530-1533.

81. Consort: Transparent Reporting of Trials. The Consort Statement. http://www.consort-statement.org/consort-statement/overview0/ . 2011.

82. Frohlich KL, Corin E, Potvin L. A theoretical proposal for the relationship between context and disease. Sociology of Health & Illness 2001;23(6):776-797.

83. Haggerty JL, Reid RJ, Freeman GK, Starfield BH, Adair CE, McKendry R. Continuity of care: a multidisciplinary review. BMJ 2003;327(7425):1219-1221.

84. Feeny D, Furlong W, Boyle M, Torrance GW. Multi-attribute health status classification systems. Health Utilities Index. Pharmacoeconomics 1995;7(6):490-502.

85. Linacre JM. Correlation Coefficients: Describing relationships. Rasch Measurement Transactions 2005;19(3):1028-1029.

86. Olsson U, Drasgaw F. The polyserial correlation coefficient. Psychometrika 1982;47:337-347.

87. Drummond MF, Sculpher MJ, Torrance GW, O'Brien BJ, Stoddart GL. Methods for the Economic Evaluation of Health Care Programmes. Third ed. Oxford Medical Publications; 2005.

88. Nunnally J, Bernstein I. Psychometric Theory. 3rd ed. New York: McGraw-Hill; 1994.

89. Eremenco SL, Cella D, Arnold BJ. A comprehensive method for the translation and cross-cultural validation of health status questionnaires. Eval Health Prof 2005;28(2):212-232.

90. Vogt WP. Dictionary of Statistics and Methodology - A Nontechnical Guide for the Social Sciences. 3rd ed. Thousand Oaks California: SAGE Publications; 2005.

91. Denzin NK, Lincoln YS. The SAGE Handbook of Qualitative Research. 4th ed. Thousand Oaks CA: SAGE Publications Inc; 2001.

92. Merriam Webster Dictionary. http://www.merriam-webster.com/ . 2012.

93. O'Connor AM, Bennett CL, Stacey D et al. Decision aids for people facing health treatment or screening decisions. Cochrane Database Syst Rev 2009;(3):CD001431.

94. O'Connor AM, Rostom A, Fiset V et al. Decision aids for patients facing health treatment or screening decisions: systematic review. BMJ 1999;319(7212):731-734.

95. Connolly T, Reb J. Regret in cancer-related decisions. Health Psychol 2005;24(4 Suppl):S29-S34.

96. Brehaut JC, O'Connor AM, Wood TJ et al. Validation of a decision regret scale. Med Decis Making 2003;23(4):281-292.

97. McKenna HP. The Delphi technique: a worthwhile research approach for nursing? J Adv Nurs 1994;19(6):1221-1225.

98. RAND. Delphi Method. http://www.rand.org/topics/delphi-method.html . 2015.

99. Keeney S, Hasson F, McKenna HP. A critical review of the Delphi technique as a research methodology for nursing. Int J Nurs Stud 2001;38(2):195-200.

100. Dalkey N, Helmer O. An experimental application of the Delphi Method to the use of experts. 1962

101. Schwartz CE, Andresen EM, Nosek MA, Krahn GL. Response shift theory: important implications for measuring quality of life in people with disability. Arch Phys Med Rehabil 2007;88(4):529-536.

102. McClimans L, Bickenbach J, Westerman M, Carlson L, Wasserman D, Schwartz C. Philosophical perspectives on response shift. Qual Life Res 2013;22(7):1871-1878.

103. Amundson R. Quality of life, disability, and hedonic psychology. Journal for the Theory of Social Behaviour 2010;40(4):374-392.

104. Blinman P, King M, Norman R, Viney R, Stockler MR. Preferences for cancer treatments: an overview of methods and applications in oncology. Ann Oncol 2012;23(5):1104-1110.

105. Nutbeam D. Health promotion glossary. Health Promotion International 1998;13(4):349-364.

106. Brozek JL, Guyatt GH, Heels-Ansdell D et al. Specific HRQL instruments and symptom scores were more responsive than preference-based generic instruments in patients with GERD. J Clin Epidemiol 2009;62(1):102-110.

107. Roberts MC, Ilardi SS. Handbook of Research Methods in Clinical Psychology. Wiley Blackwell; 2003.

108. Graham ID, Logan J, Harrison MB et al. Lost in knowledge translation: time for a map? J Contin Educ Health Prof 2006;26(1):13-24.

109. Wilson PM, Petticrew M, Calnan MW, Nazareth I. Disseminating research findings: what should researchers do? A systematic scoping review of conceptual frameworks. Implement Sci 2010;5:91.

110. Guyatt GH, Cook DJ. Health status, quality of life, and the individual. JAMA 1994;272(8):630-631.

111. Li Q, Loke AY. A literature review on the mutual impact of the spousal caregiver-cancer patients dyads: 'communication', 'reciprocal influence', and 'caregiver-patient congruence'. Eur J Oncol Nurs 2014;18(1):58-65.

112. Greenland S, Robins J. Invited commentary: ecologic studies--biases, misconceptions, and counterexamples. Am J Epidemiol 1994;139(8):747-760.

113. Chaytor N, Schmitter-Edgecombe M. The ecological validity of neuropsychological tests: a review of the literature on everyday cognitive skills. Neuropsychol Rev 2003;13(4):181-197.

114. Heaton RK, Pendleton MG. Use of Neuropsychological tests to predict adult patients' everyday functioning. J Consult Clin Psychol 1981;49(6):807-821.

115. Cohen J. Statistical power analysis for the behavioral sciences . 2nd ed. New Jersey : Lawrence Erlbaum; 1988.

116. Fritz CO, Morris PE, Richler JJ. Effect size estimates: current use, calculations, and interpretation. J Exp Psychol Gen 2012;141(1):2-18.

117. Nakagawa S, Cuthill IC. Effect size, confidence interval and statistical significance: a practical guide for biologists. Biol Rev Camb Philos Soc 2007;82(4):591-605.

118. Barbic SP, Bartlett SJ, Mayo NE. Emotional Vitality: Concept of Importance for Rehabilitation. Arch Phys Med Rehabil 2012.

119. Kubzansky LD, Thurston RC. Emotional vitality and incident coronary heart disease: benefits of healthy psychological functioning. Arch Gen Psychiatry 2007;64(12):1393-1401.

120. Webster's New World Medical Dictionary. 3 ed. Wiley; 2008.

121. Cella D. The Functional Assessment of Cancer Therapy-Anemia (FACT-An) Scale: a new tool for the assessment of outcomes in cancer anemia and fatigue. Semin Hematol 1997;34(3 Suppl 2):13-19.

122. Patrick DL, Erickson P. Health Status and Health Policy: Quality of Life in Health Care Evaluation and Resource Allocation. Oxford University Press; 1993.

123. Ryff CD. Psychological well-being revisited: advances in the science and practice of eudaimonia. Psychother Psychosom 2014;83(1):10-28.

124. Treasury Board of Canada Secretariat. Treasury Board of Canada Secretariat. http://www.tbs-sct.gc.ca/tbs-sct/index-eng.asp . 2011.

125. Centre for Evidence-Based Medicine- University of Oxford. What is Evidence-Based Medicine? http://www.cebm.net/index.aspx?o=1914 . 2009.

126. Reddel HK, Taylor DR, Bateman ED et al. An official American Thoracic Society/European Respiratory Society statement: asthma control and exacerbations: standardizing endpoints for clinical asthma trials and clinical practice. Am J Respir Crit Care Med 2009;180(1):59-99.

127. American College of Sports Medicine. ACSM's Resource Manual for Guidelines for Exercise Testing and Prescription. 6th edition ed. Baltimore, MD: Lippincott Williams & Wilkins; 2010.

128. McArdle D, Katch F, Katch V. Energy, Nutrition and Human Performance. Exercise Physiology 5th Edition ed. Baltimore, Maryland: Lipponcott Williams and Wilkins; 2001.

129. Goldstein RE. Clinical Methods: The History, Physical and Laboratory Examinations. Third Edition ed. Boston: Buttersworth; 1990.

130. Myers J, Prakash M, Froelicher V, Do D, Partington S, Atwood JE. Exercise capacity and mortality among men referred for exercise testing. N Engl J Med 2002;346(11):793-801.

131. Kaminsky DA, Knyazhitskiy A, Sadeghi A, Irvin CG. Assessing maximal exercise capacity: peak work or peak oxygen consumption? Respir Care 2014;59(1):90-96.

132. Boston P, Bruce A, Schreiber R. Existential suffering in the palliative care setting: an integrated literature review. J Pain Symptom Manage 2011;41(3):604-618.

133. Morita T, Tsunoda J, Inoue S, Chihara S. An exploratory factor analysis of existential suffering in Japanese terminally ill cancer patients. Psychooncology 2000;9(2):164-168.

134. Fairclough DL. Design and Analysis of Quality of Life Studies in Clinical Trials. Second Edition ed. Chapman & Hall/CRC; 2010.

135. Spearman C. General intelligence objectively determined and measured. American Journal of Psychology 1904;15:201-293.

136. Wilt J, Revelle W. Extraversion. In: Leary MR, Hoyle RH, editors. Handbook of Individual Differences in Social Behavior. New Yorkl: Guilford Press; 2009:27-45.

137. Paunonen SV. Big Five factors of personality and replicated predictions of behavior. J Pers Soc Psychol 2003;84(2):411-424.

138. Canadian Cancer Society. Candian Cancer Society Research Institute. http://www.cancer.ca/research/ . 2011.

139. Chaudhuri A, Behan PO. Fatigue in neurological disorders. Lancet 2004;363(9413):978-988.

140. Kluger BM, Krupp LB, Enoka RM. Fatigue and fatigability in neurologic illnesses: proposal for a unified taxonomy. Neurology 2013;80(4):409-416.

141. Fukuda K, Straus SE, Hickie I, Sharpe MC, Dobbins JG, Komaroff A. The chronic fatigue syndrome: a comprehensive approach to its definition and study. International Chronic Fatigue Syndrome Study Group. Ann Intern Med 1994;121(12):953-959.

142. Wyller VB. The chronic fatigue syndrome-an update. Acta Neurol Scand Suppl 2007;187:7-14.

143. Christley Y, Duffy T, Martin CR. A review of the definitional criteria for chronic fatigue syndrome. J Eval Clin Pract 2012;18(1):25-31.

144. Krupp LB, Alvarez LA, LaRocca NG, Scheinberg LC. Fatigue in Multiple Sclerosis. Archives of Neurology 1988;45:435-437.

145. Schoenwald SK, Garland AF, Chapman JE, Frazier SL, Sheidow AJ, Southam-Gerow MA. Toward the effective and efficient

measurement of implementation fidelity. Adm Policy Ment Health 2011;38(1):32-43.

146. Forgatch MS, Patterson GR, Degarmo DS. Evaluating fidelity: predictive validity for a measure of competent adherence to the Oregon model of parent management training. Behav Ther 2005;36(1):3-13.

147. McCrae RR, John OP. An introduction to the five-factor model and its applications. J Pers 1992;60(2):175-215.

148. McCrae RR, Costa PT, Jr. Personality trait structure as a human universal. Am Psychol 1997;52(5):509-516.

149. McDowell I. Measuring Health: A guide to rating scales and questionnaires. New York: Oxford University Press; 2006.

150. Csikszentmihalyi M. Flow: The Psychology of Optimal Experience. New York: Harper and Row; 1990.

151. Kitzinger J. Qualitative research. Introducing focus groups. BMJ 1995;311(7000):299-302.

152. Aday LA, Cornelius LJ. Designing and conducting health surveys: a comprehensive guide. John Wiley & Sons; 2011.

153. Fried LP, Ferrucci L, Darer J, Williamson JD, Anderson G. Untangling the concepts of disability, frailty, and comorbidity: implications for improved targeting and care. J Gerontol A Biol Sci Med Sci 2004;59(3):255-263.

154. Espinoza S, Walston JD. Frailty in older adults: insights and interventions. Cleve Clin J Med 2005;72(12):1105-1112.

155. Agresti A. Analysis of Ordinal Categorical Data. Hoboken NJ: Wiley; 1984.

156. Wood W, Eagly AH. Gender Identity. In: Leary MR, Hoyle RH, editors. Handbook of Individual Differences in Social Behavior. New York: Guilford Press; 2009:109-125.

157. Fougeyrollas P. Documenting environmental factors for preventing the handicap creation process: Quebec contributions relating to ICIDH and social participation of people with functional differences. Disabil Rehabil 1995;17(3-4):145-153.

158. Aristotle. Nicomachean Ethics. In: R.McKeon, editor. Introduction to Aristotle. New York: Modern Library; 1947.

159. Joshanloo M. Eastern Conceptualization of Happiness: Fundamental Differences with Western Views. Journal of Happiness Studies 2014;15:475-493.

160. Rykk CD. Happiness is Everything, or Is It? Explorations on the Meaning of Psychological Well-Being. Journal of Personality and Social Psychology 1989;57(6):1069-1081.

161. Oxford Dictionary of English. 2015. Oxford University Press.

162. World Happiness Report 2015. 2015

163. World Health Organization. Ottawa Charter for Health Promotion. Ottawa, Ontario, Canada: 1986

164. Northern & Yorkshire Public Health Observatory. An Overview of Health Impact Assessment. http://www.nepho.org.uk/publications.php5?rid=439&hl= . 2001.

165. WHO. Social Determinants of Health. http://www.who.int/social_determinants/B_132_14-en.pdf?ua=1 . 2012.

166. Kirsch I. The international Adult Literacy Survey (IALS): Understanding what was measured. Educational Testing Service, 2001RR-01-25.)

167. Kickbusch IS. Health Literacy: addressing the health and education divide. Health Promotion International 2001;16(3):289-297.

168. WHO. Regional Prepatory Meeting on Promoting Health Literacy. http://www.un.org/en/ecosoc/newfunct/pdf/chinameetinghealthliteracybackgroundpaperv2.pdf . 5-11-2009.

169. Finch E, Brooks D, Stratford PW, Mayo NE. Physical rehabilitation outcome measures. 2nd ed. Hamilton: BC Decker Inc.; 2002.

170. Davies AR, Ware JE. Measuring Health Perceptions in the Health Insurance Experiment. The Rand Corporation, 1981

171.   Donald C, Ware JE, Brook RH, Davies-Avery A. Conceptualization and measurement of health for adults in the health insurance study: Vol. IV, Social Health. Santa Monica: The Rand Corporation, 1978

172.   WHO. Budapest Declaration of Health Promotion. http://www.hphnet.org/attachments/article/40/budapes_dec.pdf . 1991.

173.   Kaplan RM. Quality of LIfe Measures: Measurement Strategies in Health Psychology. New York: John Wiley; 1985.

174.   Reid J, Wiseman-Orr ML, Scott EM, Nolan AM. Development, validation and reliability of a web-based questionnaire to measure health-related quality of life in dogs. J Small Anim Pract 2013;54(5):227-233.

175.   German AJ, Holden SL, Wiseman-Orr ML et al. Quality of life is reduced in obese dogs but improves after successful weight loss. Vet J 2012;192(3):428-434.

176.   Wiseman-Orr ML, Scott EM, Reid J, Nolan AM. Validation of a structured questionnaire as an instrument to measure chronic pain in dogs on the basis of effects on health-related quality of life. Am J Vet Res 2006;67(11):1826-1836.

177.   Wiseman-Orr ML, Nolan AM, Reid J, Scott EM. Development of a questionnaire to measure the effects of chronic pain on health-related quality of life in dogs. Am J Vet Res 2004;65(8):1077-1084.

178.   McMillan FD. Quality of life in animals. J Am Vet Med Assoc 2000;216(12):1904-1910.

179.   Dawkins MS. Animal Suffering. New York: Chapman & Hall; 1980.

180.   Gold MR, Segel JE, Russell LB, Weinstein MC. Cost-Effectiveness in Health and Medicine. New York: Oxford University Press; 1996.

181.   Spilker B. Quality of Life and Pharmacoeconomics in Clinical Trials. 2 ed. Lippincott Williams & Wilkins; 1995.

182. Norman G. Hi! How are you? Response shift, implicit theories and differing epistemologies. Qual Life Res 2003;12(3):239-249.

183. LIttle RJA, Rubin DB. Statistical Analysis with Missing Data. New York: 1987.

184. Dijkers MP. Individualization in quality of life measurement: instruments and approaches. Arch Phys Med Rehabil 2003;84(4 Suppl 2):S3-14.

185. O'Boyle CA, Hofer S, Ring L. Individualized quality of life. Assessing quality of life in clinical trials. Second ed. Oxford University Press; 2005:225-242.

186. Government of Canada. Panel on Research Ethics. Chapter 3: The Consent Process. http://www.pre.ethics.gc.ca/eng/policy-politique/initiatives/tcps2-eptc2/chapitre3-chapitre3/ . 2015.

187. WHO. Glossary of Terms for Community Health Care and Services for Older Persons. http://www.who.int/kobe_centre/ageing/ahp_vol5_glossary.pdf 5. 2004.

188. Kodner DL, Spreeuwenberg C. Integrated care: meaning, logic, applications, and implications - a discussion paper. International journal of integrated care 2002;2.

189. WHO. Innovative Care for Chronic Conditions. http://www.who.int/chp/knowledge/publications/icccreport/en/ . 2003.

190. Peduzzi P, Wittes J, Detre K, Holford T. Analysis as-randomized and the problem of non-adherence: an example from the Veterans Affairs Randomized Trial of Coronary Artery Bypass Surgery. Stat Med 1993;12(13):1185-1195.

191. Mayo NE. Randomized Trials and Other Parallel Comparisons of Treatment. In: Bailar JC, Hoaglin DC, editors. Medical Uses of Statistics. 3rd ed. Hoboken, New Jersey: A John Wiley & Sons, Inc & The New England Journal of Medicine; 2009:51-89.

192. Chang CH, Reeve BB. Item response theory and its applications to patient-reported outcomes measurement. Eval Health Prof 2005;28(3):264-282.

193. Lord FM. Applications of item response to theory to practical testing problems. Hillsdale NJ: Lawrence Erlbaum Associates; 1980.

194. Lord FM, Novick MR, Birnbaum A. Statistical theories of mental test scores. Reading MA: Addison-Wesley; 1968.

195. Chakravarty EF, Bjorner JB, Fries JF. Improving patient reported outcomes using item response theory and computerized adaptive testing. J Rheumatol 2007;34(6):1426-1431.

196. Landis JR, Koch GG. The measurement of observer agreement for categorical data. Biometrics 1977;33(1):159-174.

197. National Center for the Dissemination of Disease Research. Knowledge Translation at the Canadian Institutes of Health Research: A primer. 200718.)

198. Portney LG, Watkins MP. Foundations of Clinical Research: Applications to Practice. Conneticut: Appelton and Lange; 1993.

199. DeVellis RF. Scale Development: Theory and Application. Second ed. Sage Inc; 2003.

200. Weissman MM, Sholomskas D, Pottenger M, Prusoff BA, Locke BZ. Assessing depressive symptoms in five psychiatric populations: a validation study. Am J Epidemiol 1977;106(3):203-214.

201. Netemeyer RG, Beardon WO, Sharma S. Scaling Procedures, Issues and Applications. Thousand Oaks, CA: Sage Publications; 2003.

202. Norman GR, Streiner DL. PDQ Statistics. Third ed. BC Decker Inc; 2003.

203. Bollen KA. Latent variables in psychology and the social sciences. Annu Rev Psychol 2002;53:605-634.

204. Baker PS, Bodner EV, Allman RM. Measuring life-space mobility in community-dwelling older adults. J Am Geriatr Soc 2003;51(11):1610-1614.

205. Peel C, Sawyer BP, Roth DL, Brown CJ, Brodner EV, Allman RM. Assessing mobility in older adults: the UAB Study of Aging Life-Space Assessment. Phys Ther 2005;85(10):1008-1119.

206. DeVellis RF. Scale Development: Theory and Application. Second ed. Sage Inc; 2003.

207. Diener E, Emmons RA, Larsen RJ, Griffin S. The Satisfaction With Life Scale. J Pers Assess 1985;49(1):71-75.

208. Uebersax JS. Likert Scales: Dispelling the Confusion. http://john-uebersax.com/stat/likert.htm . 2015.

209. Armitage P, Berry G, Matthews JNS. Statistical methods in medical research. John Wiley & Sons; 2008.

210. Cramer JA, Roy A, Burrell A et al. Medication compliance and persistence: terminology and definitions. Value Health 2008;11(1):44-47.

211. Manwell LA, Barbic SP, Roberts K et al. What is mental health? Evidence towards a new definition from a mixed methods multidisciplinary international survey. BMJ Open 2015;5(6):e007079.

212. WHO. What is mental health? http://www.who.int/features/qa/62/en/ . 2007.

213. Smetanin P, Stiff D, Briante C, Adair CE, Ahmad S, Khan M. The Life and Economic Impact of Major Mental Illnesses in Canada: 2011 to 2041. Risk Analytica, on behalf of the Mental Health Commission of Canada 201, 2011

214. Mental Health Comission of Canada. 2015.

215. Systematic Reviews in Health Care: Meta-Analysis in Context. Second ed. London: BMJ Books; 2001.

216. Pai M, McCulloch M, Gorman JD et al. Systematic reviews and meta-analyses: an illustrated, step-by-step guide. Natl Med J India 2004;17(2):86-95.

217. Spiegelhalter DJ, Abrams KR, Myles JP. Bayesian Approaches to Clinical Trials and Health-Care Evaluation. 2004.

218. Li T, Puhan MA, Vedula SS, Singh S, Dickersin K. Network meta-analysis-highly attractive but more methodological research is needed. BMC Med 2011;9:79.

219. Thompson SG, Higgins JP. How should meta-regression analyses be undertaken and interpreted? Stat Med 2002;21(11):1559-1573.

220. Johnson RB, Onwuegbuzie AJ, Turner LA. Toward a definition of mixed methods research. Journal of Mixed Methods Research 2007;1(2):112-133.

221. Graham ID, Tetroe J. Some theoretical underpinnings of knowledge translation. Acad Emerg Med 2007;14(11):936-941.

222. Estabrooks CA, Thompson DS, Lovely JJ, Hofmeyer A. A guide to knowledge translation theory. J Contin Educ Health Prof 2006;26(1):25-36.

223. Wilson IB, Cleary PD. Linking clinical variables with health-related quality of life. A conceptual model of patient outcomes. JAMA 1995;273(1):59-65.

224. Andrich D. Rating scales and Rasch measurement. Expert Rev Pharmacoecon Outcomes Res 2011;11(5):571-585.

225. Cano S, Klassen AF, Scott A, Thoma A, Feeny D, Pusic A. Health outcome and economic measurement in breast cancer surgery: challenges and opportunities. Expert Rev Pharmacoecon Outcomes Res 2010;10(5):583-594.

226. Rubin DB. Multiple imputation for nonresponse in surveys. New York: Wiley; 1987.

227. McAlister FA, Clark HD, van WC et al. The medical review article revisited: has the science improved? Ann Intern Med 1999;131(12):947-951.

228. Hawe P, Webster C, Shiell A. A glossary of terms for navigating the field of social network analysis. J Epidemiol Community Health 2004;58(12):971-975.

229. Gallagher M, Hares T, Spencer J, Bradshaw C, Webb I. The nominal group technique: a research tool for general practice? Fam Pract 1993;10(1):76-81.

230. Delbecq AL, VandeVen AH. A Group Process Model for Problem Identification and Program Planning. Journal of Applied Behavioral Science 1971;VII:466-491.

231. Business Dictionary. 2015.

232. D'Agostino RB, Sr., Massaro JM, Sullivan LM. Non-inferiority trials: design concepts and issues - the encounters of academic consultants in statistics. Stat Med 2003;22(2):169-186.

233. Kleinbaum DG, Kupper LL, Muller KE. Applied regression analysis and other multivariable methods. Boston: PWS-KENT Publishing Co.; 1988.

234. Zermansky A. Number needed to harm should be measured for treatments. BMJ 1998;317(7164):1014.

235. Hjermstad MJ, Fayers PM, Haugen DF et al. Studies comparing Numerical Rating Scales, Verbal Rating Scales, and Visual Analogue Scales for assessment of pain intensity in adults: a systematic literature review. J Pain Symptom Manage 2011;41(6):1073-1093.

236. Townsend EA, Polatajko HJ. Enabling Occupation II: Advancing an occupational therpay vision for health, well-being & justice through occupation. 2nd ed. Ottawa: CAOT; 2013.

237. McCrae RR, Costa PT, Jr. Conceptions and Correlates of Openness to Experience. In: Hogan R, Johnson J, editors. Handbook of Personality Psychology. Orlando FL: Academic Press; 1997:825-842.

238. McCrae RR, Sutin AR. Openness to Experience. In: Leary MR, Hoyle RH, editors. Handbook of Individual Differences in Social Behavior. New York: Guilford Press; 2009:257-273.

239. Hennekens CH, Buring JE. Epidemiology in Medicine. 1st ed. Boston: Little, Brown and Company; 1987.

240. Scott S, Goldberg M, Mayo N. Statistical Assessment of ordinal outcomes in comparative studies. Journal of Clinical Epidemiology 1997;50:45-55.

241. White KL. Improved medical care statistics and the health services system. Public Health Rep 1967;82(10):847-854.

242. Bailar JC, Hoaglin DC. Medical Uses in Statistics. 3 ed. Wiley; 2009.

243. Higgins J, Mayo NE, Desrosiers J, Salbach NM, Ahmed S. Upper extremity function and recovery in the acute phase post stroke. J Rehabil Res Dev. In press.

244. Macaulay AC, Commanda LE, Freeman WL et al. Participatory research maximises community and lay involvement. North American Primary Care Research Group. BMJ 1999;319(7212):774-778.

245. Institute of Medicine. Crossing the quality chasm: A new health system for the 21st century. Washington: National Academy Press; 2001.

246. Frank L, Basch E, Selby JV. The PCORI perspective on patient-centered outcomes research. JAMA 2014;312(15):1513-1514.

247. Rathert C, Wyrwich MD, Boren SA. Patient-centered care and outcomes: a systematic review of the literature. Med Care Res Rev 2013;70(4):351-379.

248. PCORI. Patient-Centered Outcomes. http://www.pcori.org/research-we-support/pcor/ . 2012.

249. Frank L, Forsythe L, Ellis L et al. Conceptual and practical foundations of patient engagement in research at the patient-centered outcomes research institute. Qual Life Res 2015;24(5):1033-1041.

250. The HCAHPS Survey:Frequently Asked Questions. http://www cms gov/Medicare/Quality-Initiatives-Patient-Assessment-Instruments/HospitalQualityInits/Downloads/HospitalHCAHPSFactSheet201007 pdf, 2015http://www.cms.gov/Medicare/Quality-Initiatives-Patient-Assessment-

Instruments/HospitalQualityInits/Downloads/HospitalHCAHP
SFactSheet201007.pdf).

251. Ross CK, Frommelt G, Hazelwood L, Chang RW. The role of
      expectations in patient satisfaction with medical care. J
      Health Care Mark 1987;16-26.

252. Bjertnaes OA, Sjetne IS, Iversen HH. Overall patient
      satisfaction with hospitals: effects of patient-reported
      experiences and fulfilment of expectations. BMJ Qual Saf
      2012;21(1):39-46.

253. Ware JE, Jr., Davies-Avery A, Stewart AL. The measurement
      and meaning of patient satisfaction. Health Med Care Serv
      Rev 1978;1(1):1, 3-1,15.

254. Picker Institute. Improving healthcare through the patient's
      eyes: Principles of patient-centered care.
      http://pickerinstitute.org/ . 2015.

255. Mayo NE, Figueiredo S. Measuring what Matters: What's in a
      Name? Journal of Clinical Epidemiology 2015.

256. Department of Health and Human Services. Healthy People
      2020: An Opportunity to Address Societal Determinants of
      Health in the US.
      http://www.healthypeople.gov/2020/about/advisory/Societ
      alDeterminantsHealth.pdf . 2010.

257. Everitt B. Medical Statistics from A to Z: a guide for clinicans.
      Cambridge: 2006.

258. Leon AC, Davis LL, Kraemer HC. The role and interpretation
      of pilot studies in clinical research. J Psychiatr Res
      2011;45(5):626-629.

259. Bearman JE, Loewenson RB, Gullen WH. Muench's
      postulates,laws, and corollaries, or biometricians' views of
      clinical studies. Biometrics 1974;Note No. 4 (April).

260. Figueiredo S, Mayo NE. What pilot studies tell us! Disabil
      Rehabil 2015;1-2.

261. Sackett DL, Cook DJ. Can we learn anything from small trials?
      Ann N Y Acad Sci 1993;703:25-31.

262. Cronbach LJ, Ambron SR, Dornbusch SM et al. Toward reform of program evaluation: aims, methods, and institutional arrangements. San Fransisco CA: Jossey-Bass; 1980.

263. Shapiro AK, Shapiro E. The Powerful Placebo: From Ancient Priest to Modern Physician. JHU Press; 2000.

264. Berry SM, Connor JT, Lewis RJ. The platform trial: an efficient strategy for evaluating multiple treatments. JAMA 2015;313(16):1619-1620.

265. Rothman KJ, Greenland S, Lash T. Modern Epidemiology. 3 ed. Lippincott, Williams and Wilkinson; 2008.

266. Mayo NE. Understanding Analyses of Randomized Trials. In: Bailar JC, Hoaglin DC, editors. Medical Uses of Statistics. 3rd ed. Hoboken, New Jersey: A John Wiley & Sons, Inc & The New England Journal of Medicine; 2009:195-237.

267. Mayo NE, Wood-Dauphinee S, Cote R et al. There's no place like home: an evaluation of early supported discharge for stroke. Stroke 2000;31(5):1016-1023.

268. Weinstein MC, Torrance G, McGuire A. QALYs: the basics. Value Health 2009;12 Suppl 1:S5-S9.

269. Gold M, Franks P, Erickson P. Assessing the health of the nation. The predictive validity of a preference-based measure and self-rated health. Med Care 1996;34(2):163-177.

270. Revicki DA, Leidy NK, Brennan-Diemer F, Sorensen S, Togias A. Integrating patient preferences into health outcomes assessment: the multiattribute Asthma Symptom Utility Index. Chest 1998;114(4):998-1007.

271. Dolan P. Whose preferences count? Med Decis Making 1999;19(4):482-486.

272. Iliffe S. Medication review for older people in general practice. J R Soc Med 1994;87 Suppl 23:11-13.

273. Onder G, van der Cammen TJ, Petrovic M, Somers A, Rajkumar C. Strategies to reduce the risk of iatrogenic illness in complex older adults. Age Ageing 2013;42(3):284-291.

274. WHO. Primary Health Care. http://www.unicef.org/about/history/files/Alma_Ata_confer ence_1978_report.pdf . 1978.

275. Hebel JR, McCarter RJ. Study Guide to Epidemiology and Biostatistics. 6 ed. Jones and Bartlett Publishing; 2006.

276. Rosenbaum P, Rubin D. The central role of the propensity score in observational studies for causal effects. Biometrika 1983;70:41-55.

277. D'Agostino RB, Jr. Propensity score methods for bias reduction in the comparison of a treatment to a non-randomized control group. Stat Med 1998;17(19):2265-2281.

278. Williamson EJ, Forbes A. Introduction to propensity scores. Respirology 2014;19(5):625-635.

279. Friedman GD. Primer of Epidemiology. 4 ed. USA: 1994.

280. Michell J. Measurement in Psychology: A critical history of methodological concept. United Kingdom: Cambridge Press; 1999.

281. Patrick DL, Curtis JR, Engelberg RA, Nielsen E, McCown E. Measuring and improving the quality of dying and death. Ann Intern Med 2003;139(5 Pt 2):410-415.

282. Approaching Death: Improving care at the end of life. Washington: National Academy Press; 1997.

283. Stewart AL, Teno J, Patrick DL, Lynn J. The concept of quality of life of dying persons in the context of health care. J Pain Symptom Manage 1999;17(2):93-108.

284. Flanagan JC. A research approach to improve our quality of life. American Psychologist 1978;33:138-147.

285. Flanagan JC. Measurement of quality of life: current state of the art. Arch Phys Med Rehabil 1982;63(2):56-59.

286. The World Health Organization Quality of Life assessment (WHOQOL): position paper from the World Health Organization. Soc Sci Med 1995;41(10):1403-1409.

287. Gill TM, Feinstein AR. A critical appraisal of the quality of quality-of-life measurements. JAMA 1994;272(8):619-626.

288. Farm Animal Welfare Coumcil. FAWC updates the five freedoms. Veterinary Record 1992;131:357.

289. Wojciechowska JI, Hewson CJ. Quality-of-life assessment in pet dogs. J Am Vet Med Assoc 2005;226(5):722-728.

290. Taylor KD, Mills DS. Is quality of life a useful concept for companion animals? Animal Welfare 2007;16:55-65.

291. Elandt-Johnson RC. Definition of rates: some remarks on their use and misuse. Am J Epidemiol 1975;102(4):267-271.

292. Rosenburg L, Joseph L, Barkun A. Surgical Arithmetic: Epidemiological, Statistical and Outcome-Based Approach to Surgical Practice. Georgetown Texas, USA: Landes Bioscience; 2000.

293. Anthony WA. Recovery from mental illness: the guiding vision of the mental health service system in the 1990's. Pyschosocial Rehabilitation Journal 1993;16(4):11-23.

294. Mental Health Commission of Canada. Changing directions, changing lives: The mental health strategy for Canada. Calgary AB: 2012

295. Canadian Mental Health Association. Recovery. https://ontario.cmha.ca/mental-health/mental-health-conditions/recovery/ . 2015.

296. Allvin R, Berg K, Idvall E, Nilsson U. Postoperative recovery: a concept analysis. J Adv Nurs 2007;57(5):552-558.

297. Meyer T, Gutenbrunner C, Bickenbach J, Cieza A, Melvin J, Stucki G. Towards a conceptual description of rehabilitation as a health strategy. J Rehabil Med 2011;43(9):765-769.

298. Nici L, Donner C, Wouters E et al. American Thoracic Society/European Respiratory Society statement on pulmonary rehabilitation. Am J Respir Crit Care Med 2006;173(12):1390-1413.

299. Gamble GL, Gerber LH, Spill GR, Paul KL. The future of cancer rehabilitation: emerging subspecialty. Am J Phys Med Rehabil 2011;90(5 Suppl 1):S76-S87.

300. Figueiredo S, Finch L, Mai J, Ahmed S, Huang A, Mayo NE. Nordic walking for geriatric rehabilitation: a randomized pilot trial. Disabil Rehabil 2013;35(12):968-975.

301. Balducci L, Fossa SD. Rehabilitation of older cancer patients. Acta Oncol 2013;52(2):233-238.

302. Leidy NK. Using functional status to assess treatment outcomes. Chest 1994;106(6):1645-1646.

303. Nucci M, Mapelli D, Mondini S. Cognitive Reserve Index questionnaire (CRIq): a new instrument for measuring cognitive reserve. Aging Clin Exp Res 2012;24(3):218-226.

304. Dyrbye LN, Power DV, Massie FS et al. Factors associated with resilience to and recovery from burnout: a prospective, multi-institutional study of US medical students. Med Educ 2010;44(10):1016-1026.

305. Nemeth C, Wears R, Woods D, Hollnagel E, Cook R. Minding the Gaps: Creating Resilience in Health Care. 2008.

306. Windle G, Bennett KM, Noyes J. A methodological review of resilience measurement scales. Health Qual Life Outcomes 2011;9:8.

307. Windle G. The Resilience Network: What is resilience? A systematic review and concept analysis. Reviews in Clinical Gerontology 2010;21:1-18.

308. Schwartz CE, Sprangers MAG. Adaptation to Changing Health response shift in Quality-of-Life Research. 1st ed. Washington, DC: American Psychological Association; 2000.

309. Barclay-Goddard R, Epstein JD, Mayo NE. Response shift: a brief overview and proposed research priorities. Qual Life Res 2009;18(3):335-346.

310. Arksey H, O'Malley L. Scoping studies: towards a methodological framework. International Journal of Social Research Methodology 2005;8(1):19-32.

311. WHO. Violence against women. http://www.who.int/mediacentre/factsheets/fs239/en/ . 2013.

312. Roberts JS, Uhlmann WR. Genetic susceptibility testing for neurodegenerative diseases: ethical and practice issues. Prog Neurobiol 2013;110:89-101.

313. Boulos MN, Hetherington L, Wheeler S. Second Life: an overview of the potential of 3-D virtual worlds in medical and health education. Health Info Libr J 2007;24(4):233-245.

314. Bandura A. Self-efficacy: The exercise of control. New York: W.H. Freeman; 1997.

315. Stanford School of Medicine. Stanford Small-Group Self-Management Programs in English. http://patienteducation.stanford.edu/programs/ . 2014.

316. Expert Patients Programme. http://www.expertpatients.co.uk/ . 2014.

317. Flinders University. The Flinders Program. http://www.flinders.edu.au/medicine/sites/fhbhru/self-management.cfm . 2014.

318. Barlow J, Wright C, Sheasby J, Turner A, Hainsworth J. Self-management approaches for people with chronic conditions: a review. Patient Educ Couns 2002;48(2):177-187.

319. Lorig KR, Sobel DS, Stewart AL et al. Evidence suggesting that a chronic disease self-management program can improve health status while reducing hospitalization: a randomized trial. Med Care 1999;37(1):5-14.

320. Clark NM, Becker MH, Janz NK, Lorig K, Rakowski W, Anderson L. Self-Management of Chronic Disease by Older Adults: A Review and Questions for Research. Journal of Aging Health 1991;3:3-27.

321. Mossey JM, Shapiro E. Self-rated health: a predictor of mortality among the elderly. Am J Public Health 1982;72(8):800-808.

322. Layes A, Asada Y, Kepart G. Whiners and deniers - what does self-rated health measure? Soc Sci Med 2012;75(1):1-9.

323. Mantzavinis GD, Pappas N, Dimoliatis ID, Ioannidis JP. Multivariate models of self-reported health often neglected

essential candidate determinants and methodological issues. J Clin Epidemiol 2005;58(5):436-443.

324. Rosenzveig A, Kuspinar A, Daskalopoulou SS, Mayo NE. Toward patient-centered care: a systematic review of how to ask questions that matter to patients. Medicine (Baltimore) 2014;93(22):e120.

325. Bowling A. Just one question: If one question works, why ask several? J Epidemiol Community Health 2005;59(5):342-345.

326. Barlow DH, Nock MK, Hersen M. Single Case Experimental Designs: Strategies for Studying Behavior Change. Third Edition ed. Pearson Education Inc.; 2009.

327. Crowne DP, Marlowe D. A new scale of social desirability independent of psychopathology. J Consult Psychol 1960;24:349-354.

328. Dillman DA. Mail and Telephone Surveys: The Total Design method. New York: Don Wiley & Son; 1978.

329. Levasseur M, Richard L, Gauvin L, Raymond E. Inventory and analysis of definitions of social participation found in the aging literature: proposed taxonomy of social activities. Soc Sci Med 2010;71(12):2141-2149.

330. Le Réseau international sur le Processus de production du handicap (RIPPH). La participation Sociale. http://www.ripph.qc.ca . 2015.

331. Isaksson AK, Ahlstrom G. Managing chronic sorrow: experiences of patients with multiple sclerosis. J Neurosci Nurs 2008;40(3):180-191.

332. Muennig P. Cost-Effectiveness Analysis in Health: A Practical Approach. 2 ed. San Francisco, CA: Jossey-Bass; 2008.

333. Brown CA, Lilford RJ. The stepped wedge trial design: a systematic review. BMC Med Res Methodol 2006;6:54.

334. Mdege ND, Man MS, Taylor Nee Brown CA, Torgerson DJ. Systematic review of stepped wedge cluster randomized trials shows that design is particularly used to evaluate interventions during routine implementation. J Clin Epidemiol 2011;64(9):936-948.

335. Romney DM, Evans DR. Toward a general model of health-related quality of life. Qual Life Res 1996;5(2):235-241.

336. Mayo N, Asano M. Not another meta-analysis! Mult Scler 2009;15(4):409-411.

337. Moher D, Liberati A, Tetzlaff J, Altman DG. Preferred reporting items for systematic reviews and meta-analyses: the PRISMA statement. J Clin Epidemiol 2009;62(10):1006-1012.

338. National Multiple Sclerosis Society. http://www nationalmssociety org/index aspx, 2012http://www.nationalmssociety.org/index.aspx).

339. Green S, Higgins JPT, Alderson P, Clarke M, Mulrow CD, Oxman AD. Introduction. In: Higgins JPT, Green S, editors. Cochrane Handbook for Systematic reviews of Intervention. version 5.1.0. The Cochrane Collaboration; 2011.

340. Barclay-Goddard R, King J, Dubouloz CJ, Schwartz CE. Building on transformative learning and response shift theory to investigate health-related quality of life changes over time in individuals with chronic health conditions and disability. Arch Phys Med Rehabil 2012;93(2):214-220.

341. Conway K, Acquadro C, Patrick DL. Usefulness of translatability assessment: results from a retrospective study. Qual Life Res 2014;23(4):1199-1210.

342. Walton MK, Powers JH, Patrick DL et al. Clinical Outcome Assessments: Conceptual Foundation. Value in Health. In press.

343. WHO. Health Systems Financing: The Path to Universal Coverage. http://www.who.int/whr/2010/en/ . 2010.

344. Fishburn PC. Utilty Theory. Management Science 1968;14(5).

345. Messick S. Validity of psychological assessment: validation of inferences from persons' responses and performances as scientific inquiry into score meaning. American Psychologist 1995;50(9):741.

346. Dolan P, Sutton M. Mapping visual analogue scale health state valuations onto standard gamble and time trade-off values. Soc Sci Med 1997;44(10):1519-1530.

347. Sikula A Sr., Costa AD. Are Women More Ethical than Men? Journal of Business Ethics 1994;13:859-871.

348. Kitwood T. Cognition and Emotion in the Pschology of Human Values. Oxford Review of Education 1984;10(3):293-301.

349. Emerson J, Wachowicz J, Chun S. Social Return on Investment (SROI): Exploring Aspects of Value Creation. 29-1-2001.

350. EuroQol Group. EQ-5D: A standardised instrument for use as a measure of health outcome. http://www.euroqol.org/eq-5d/what-is-eq-5d/eq-5d-nomenclature.html . 2011.

351. Barak A, Klein B, Proudfoot JG. Defining internet-supported therapeutic interventions. Ann Behav Med 2009;38(1):4-17.

352. Bullinger M, Anderson R, Cella D, Aaronson N. Developing and Evaluating Cross-Cultural Instruments from Minimum Requirements to Optimal Models. Quality of Life Research 1993;2(6):451-459.

353. Tessier A, Zavorsky GS, Kim dJ, Carli F, Christou N, Mayo NE. Understanding the Determinants of Weight-Related Quality of Life among Bariatric Surgery Candidates. J Obes 2012;2012.

354. Ryff CD, Singer B. Psychological well-being: meaning, measurement, and implications for psychotherapy research. Psychother Psychosom 1996;65(1):14-23.

355. Wilson IB, Cleary PD. Linking clinical variables with health-related quality of life. A conceptual model of patient outcomes. Journal of the American Medical Association 1995;273(1):59-65.

www.ingramcontent.com/pod-product-compliance
Lightning Source LLC
Chambersburg PA
CBHW072133020426
42334CB00018B/1775